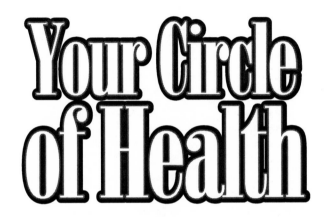

Your Circle of Health

A Holistic Reference Guide to Natural Health

Susan A. Hall, RN, ND, PhD

ISBN: 978-1-929661-36-7

Library of Congress Control Number: 2010934738

Unattributed quotations are by Susan A. Hall

Copyright © Susan A. Hall

Illustrator: William Hall

Editor: Karen Jean Bennett

Coeditors: Marjorie Reynolds, William Hall, Frank Jirmasek, Helen Jirmasek, Jane Henkles

Sample Hair Analysis by permission of Trace Elements, Inc.

Cover: Mark Lorenzo

First printing, first edition: September, 2010
Second printing, Revised first edition, March 2011

Transpersonal Publishing, div. AHU,LLC
PO Box 7220, Kill Devil Hills, NC 27948
www.TranspersonalPublishing.com
800-296-MIND

Transpersonal Publishing is a "green publisher." Most books are printed on recycled paper (look for the recycle symbol on the cover). All titles and distributed lines are available at special quantity discounts for bulk purchases for conferences/conventions, fund-raising, and educational or institutional use. For details, contact the publisher.

Authors seeking a publisher must submit query letters by e-mail to have their work considered, and only through the submission guidelines on the website.

Orders:
Email: Orders@holistictree.com
Wholesale—www.TranspersonalPublishing.com; or phone the publisher
Retail—www.Holistictree.com; go to the online shopping cart

Printed in the USA on FSC certified, recycled paper.

CONTENTS

AUTHOR'S BACKGROUND

Education and Certification

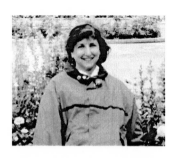

Received Registered Nurse (RN) degree in 1974

Earned Master's Degrees in Nursing (MN) and Health Services Administration (MHSA).

Certification as a Developmental Disability Nurse (CDDN)

Palliative Care Certification (end-of-life care)

National Health Care Quality Certification (CPHQ)

Certified Case Manager (CCM)

Naturopathic Doctorate (ND) in 2007

PhD in Natural Health in 2010

Clinical Background and Experience

Eleven years in home health care – Visiting Nurse Association, Director of Extended Care for professionals and paraprofessionals, staffing shift work in homes of medically fragile patients

Twenty-seven years in hospitals/LTAC - orthopedics, obstetrics, high-risk nursery, medical/ surgical, intensive care, cardiac care, risk management, quality assurance.

Acting Executive Director and Director of Nursing for St. Elizabeth Anne Seton Acute Care Hospital

Eight years as Certified Developmental Disabilities Nurse working with the developmentally disabled at ResCare

Member of the Board of Directors at American Holistic University, (AHU)

DEDICATION

I dedicate this book to my husband, William; brother Allen; mom, Jane; dad, Al; and my dear friend and editor, Karen. All of those persons encouraged me to look beyond what I have already learned and to be open to more possibilities. This hit home for me when I lost my mother who died from a stroke on April 17, 2006. I wondered if more could have been done to help her through nontraditional, natural health care methods.

The book cover design colors are dedicated to my Godchild Nathan Chips who died at a young age of 19 on 2/14/09.

ACKNOWLEDGEMENTS

Special Thanks

Thank you to my husband, William, children, Jamie and Christopher, and to my extended family who understood my passion to learn, and who supported me in this endeavor.

I also want to thank my brother, Allen Chips, DCH., PhD, and his wife, Dee Chips, BSW., M.Ht., C.R.M., for opening my mind to integrative methods in health care and for starting me in this direction through my studies at American Holistic University.

Thanks to my friends, Helen Jirmasek, ND and Frank Jirmasek, Karen and Wayne, Jan, Sheila, and Joyce who also volunteered to participate in my study.

DISCLAIMER

This book provides alternative health care options and education about living a healthy lifestyle.

It is essential for you to understand that practitioners of natural health do not diagnose, assist in treatment, or claim to cure illnesses. We educate and offer suggested nutritional programs and other complementary health care options for improving overall health and physical fitness.

Doctors of Naturopathy (ND) are licensed in 11 states. I do not function as a physician, diagnose or treat disease, nor do my services or suggestions replace the necessary services of a licensed physician.

It is your right to be informed and to choose what is best for you. Whatever your choices are, you assume responsibility for risks and you should coordinate all options with your professional health care practitioners. The publisher, the author, and their treatment centers, testimonies, and organizations discussed in this book assume no responsibility for personal health care choices.

To protect privacy, some names of my health care providers, and most of the clients' names, have been changed in this book, except where permission was granted or their stories were in the public domain.

I have not received any funding or sponsorship from any person or entity to promote this book, nor have any clients whose testimonials appear here.

"Spirit is the life, mind is the builder, and the physical is the result."[1]

Edgar Cayce

INTRODUCTION

The purpose of this book is to provide a quick reference guide to alternative and complementary natural health care options from popular health approaches. It would be time-consuming and expensive for you to gather information from all the natural health care resources available. This book will give you the flavor of those natural alternative health care remedy books and it will highlight their contents. Within this guide, there are sometimes-differing opinions on how the foods we eat, process, and eliminate, affect our physical body systems. Those factors, in turn, influence our overall health and physical and mental well-being. I am not advocating one method over another. I am merely compiling different authors' opinions on what natural remedies they think are best and presenting them as an intertwining circle of health. Remember, the goal is to guide you on your circle of health, and to assist you in achieving quality of life through healthy choices.

A thorough assessment from a reputable naturopathic doctor (ND) can help you choose what is best for your body based on your lifestyle and responses during the evaluation.

The first circle of health incorporates nutrition and exercise, or, as we think of it, our physical body.

The second circle of health is mental health, or our emotions, inner thoughts, and inner light. Those emotions and thoughts also affect the way we eat. Stress is a major component of our emotions and it, ultimately, affects our eating habits.

The final circle of health, which is interwoven with the other circles, is spiritual health, or our values and beliefs. All of those circles overlap and influence the way we make choices about our health and the results that follow.

The following questions test your awareness of other integrative health care options:

1. Are prescribed medications and surgery the most common choices for healing illness and disease?

2. Does blood type influence the immune system's responses to foods and illnesses?

3. Do herbs, supplements, acupressure, chiropractics, aromatherapy, applied kinesiology, chelation therapy, hypnotherapy and biofeedback have a place in your body's fight against illnesses?

4. Can food selection alter urine and saliva pH, and thus affect your health?

5. Does eating proteins (meat) and starches (potatoes) together at a meal affect your health?

If you answered NO to any of those questions, the information gained from this material will enlighten you about different options available, especially how choices in nutrition affect your circle of health.

"The Physical is the Result..." [1]
~Edgar Cayce

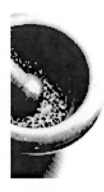

PART ONE

FIRST CIRCLE OF HEALTH
Physical Health: Nutrition and Exercise

The first six chapters present different viewpoints on nutrition, supplements, acid/alkaline foods, blood type food selections, food combinations, and exercise. Some concepts may seem extreme and may be difficult to achieve with your present lifestyle. This quick reference guide aids in finding basic information without having to buy, borrow, and read numerous resources. The concepts that fit your personal lifestyle and health condition can then be applied.

CHAPTER I

Testimonial on Nutrition and Herbal Remedies

Patsy Reynolds, ND, [2] has been involved with natural health care for over 15 years. I met her in 2007 during my internship for my naturopathic doctorate degree. Her formal education began through Nature's Sunshine[3] seminars and certification through the National Association of Certified Natural Health Professionals classes. Nature's Sunshine emphasizes education and carries pure herbs and essential oils. Their focus is on nutrition and supplements as part of food processing and elimination for the body's systems, glands, and organs to function efficiently.

Dr. Reynolds recommended the above classes in addition to study at a reputable university in naturopathic medicine for the doctorate level. One such on-line university is American Holistic University (AHU).[4] It offers a variety of courses and degrees in natural health care. Another useful resource is the American Association of Drugless Practitioners, an association for continuing education in integrative options. In addition to recommending supplements, Dr. Reynolds also emphasized that learning from one another (networking) is vital, and she also suggested www.pureherbs.com[5] that car-

2

ries pure essential oils.

While I was working with Dr. Reynolds at Mann's Harbor, North Carolina, she shared different modalities available for assisting clients. She noted that there is not just one method of care,(traditional medicine) that contains all the answers. Dr. Reynolds first became aware of alternative health care options in 1987. In 1993, at age 50, very ill and crippled with arthritis, she became aware of alternative health care options.

Dr. Reynolds, who is also a retired nurse, had tried all types of traditional medicine to treat her arthritis, to no avail. *"We were taught to trust our medical doctors as 'all knowing' and to do as they say. Over the years, people realize they are as human as the next person and they do the best they can with drugs, etc.,"* she said. She added that some doctors learn, while others become afraid to explore other options.

Some medical doctors have told Dr. Reynolds that part of their training in medical school included ordering diagnostic tests - often without conducting a physical exam or waiting until labs and x-rays were completed - and automatically ordering at least three prescriptions, whether or not they were needed. Without those prescriptions, doctors told her, clients had no confidence in them. Not all medical schools teach in that manner. Knowledge of such practice helps us understand the pressure doctors experience because of public expectations. "They are between a rock and a hard place," Dr. Reynolds said. According to her, the current overuse of antibiotics with the resulting resistive "bugs" is a good example of that practice. Medical students also have shared with Dr. Reynolds that they are told to give blood thinners to clients who are 60 and older, and they should stay on those medications for the rest of their lives. Synthetic blood thinners, such as Coumadin, have been known to cause hair loss and to impede healing. Dr. Reynolds says that herbal formulas are available to "thin" the blood, eliminating the need for synthetic blood thinners.

Much has also been written about pharmaceutical companies and the American Medical Association that profit inordinately from illnesses by utilizing strong lobbyists in government. Although that concept is not further addressed in this book, it is important to acknowledge all factors that affect your health care choices. See Additional Resources that pertain to this issue.

Dr. Reynolds' referrals have been from word-of-mouth, from medical doctors who know her, and from clients who have been helped through her integrative methods. Most of her focus is on lifestyle changes, diet, natural remedies, and supplements.

When accepting clients, Dr. Reynolds first gathers a complete medical history, concentrating on the last five years. Once the medical history is reviewed, she explores further using other integrated methods, which include a history of nutrition based on acid-alkaline foods, food combinations, blood type, muscle testing, iridology, herbs, essential oils, and flower remedies (homeopathic), and by evaluating remedies through applied kinesiology with the client. The client has to agree to work with her for 90 days, and to comply with the nutrition and supplement regimens she recommends.

Some of the tools she uses include ear candling; acupressure; Chi machine; ionic footbaths; a Rife machine on frequencies (which aids clients with Lyme's disease and many other concerns), and a parasite zapper. Dr. Reynolds stated she also used supplements from Nature's Sunshine and Pure Herbs Company, a company with the highest and purest quality herbal supplements, as opposed to synthetic products. According to Dr. Reynolds, our bodies do not always assimilate synthetic supplements.

The effects of certain food combinations were also discussed by Dr. Reynolds, such as protein (meat) and starches (potatoes) combined, and sugar and starches combined. She said those items should not be combined at one meal, especially if the client has very poor digestion. This concept will be discussed later in this book. It was one of the main areas that she changed in her personal meal planning. Almost all of her clients have responded well to her recommendations and, through their positive results, many members of her community have sought her help.

Dr. Reynolds shared many tips about when to eat certain foods and the use of supplements that aided in her turnaround. She said that when she first decided to begin her recovery process, she was extremely debilitated. Her husband had to carry her to the sofa. She said that she was in severe pain and, when anyone touched her mattress while she was on it, shocks permeated her body.

Dr. Reynolds said she was watching a natural health program on food combinations on television when she decided she should try that method since nothing else had worked. She studied the digestion times and combinations of certain types of foods. For example, fruit is best eaten in the morning, she claimed, and takes two to three hours to digest. Caffeinated coffee in the morning is acceptable, she added, but it is a diuretic that can cause the body to dehydrate. A decaffeinated product does not function as a diuretic. It is also best, Dr. Reynolds said, to fresh-grind any type of coffee and drink it within 20 minutes. All coffee is highly acidic. But kukicha twig tea6 is alkaline, and drinking it immediately after coffee assists in neutralization. The ideal acid –alkaline food balance she advocates will be further discussed later in this book.

Dr. Reynolds found that beverages should not be taken with meals. Beverages dilute the stomach's hydrochloric acid that is needed for digestion. Consuming liquids fifteen minutes prior to a meal and waiting one hour after a meal is recommended. For someone with a compromised digestive system, waiting two hours after a meal before ingesting liquids is recommended. Pure water is the preferred liquid, she claimed. Flavored waters may contain aspartame or sucrolose, such as NutraSweet and Splenda products, and cause an acidic pH level that can compromise good health.

To heal herself, Dr. Reynolds said she avoided combining starches and proteins at the same meal, as well as starches and sugars. She offered suggestions to help with selecting foods. It is best to have starches and vegetables at lunch and protein (meat) with vegetables at supper. If possible, she explained, eat fresh, raw or steamed vegetables. Meat usually takes up to 12 hours to digest and can linger in the colon for up to three days.

Pasteurized cow's milk takes up to 12 hours to digest. It is best taken at night, by itself, if at all. If milk is needed, she suggested switching to soy or a form of nut milk. Almond milk is more alkaline and also has a nice taste. Dr. Reynolds noted that milk products do cause mucous.

Bacon and eggs, which are protein, also take up to 12 hours to digest. Dr. Reynolds recommended no toast with meat protein foods. Toast is a starch that takes up to five hours to digest, and should not be combined with protein. Butter is a fat, but also an alkaline if not cooked, and can take up to12 hours to digest, she said. Most oils and butter should be eaten with the evening meal. It allows the body to process until the next meal in the morning, according to Dr. Reynolds.

Dr. Reynolds recommended fresh fruits only at breakfast, since they take two to three hours to digest. She stated that sugars were not to be combined with starches. Pure sugar is not good for the body because it is very acidic. Honey, maple syrup, or unbleached cane sugars are better but still slightly acidic. Stevia is a good, natural, sweet supplement and it contains chromium.

Dr. Reynolds said that MSG, which is in almost all food products, has been found to create cravings in clients. She said that it is a clinical problem in diets.

Once Dr. Reynolds consumed protein, she did not need it again for another 12 hours. She also added that hard-shelled fish like lobster, crab, and shrimp are all bottom feeders, and are full of toxins. Those types of fish should rarely be eaten, if at all, according to her.

An important supplement is Probiotics Eleven, a form of good bacteria available through Nature's Sunshine, Dr. Reynolds said. This bacteria is needed all the time and, especially, while on antibiotics. On her road to recovery, Dr. Reynolds said she fortified her diet with Probiotics and enzymes, vitamins, and mineral supplements.

By changing how she combined foods and by learning how the body digests certain food types, Dr. Reynolds said her body began to detoxify. Unwanted toxins containing excess protein from foods eaten were expelled. She had been bedridden and crippled from joint contractions but she slowly began to see her body respond positively. Her joints became less contracted and, soon, she was able to walk again. She also lost nine pounds the first week using combining foods properly.

Believing arthritis to be a digestive disease, Dr. Reynolds began assessing information on food combinations and food groups. She learned that blood type also affects one's physical response to food. Her resource for this information was Eat Right 4 Your Blood Type by Peter D'Adamo.[7] Those two areas will be addressed later in more detail.

Dr. Reynolds told of another client profoundly affected by altering food combinations and taking supplements. This client was on insulin and her body was getting worse. Her medical doctor said not much more could be done for her besides regulating insulin based on her diabetic diet. Through a gentle colon cleansing over 30 days and by working with different food combinations (avoiding mixing protein and starch, and sugar and starch), this client experienced a miraculous turnaround. Her physician was able to wean her from insulin. She now takes supplemental enzymes and other supplements.

The next chapter will explore acid-alkaline foods and the effects on your urine and saliva pH.

CHAPTER II

PH Testing and Acid-Alkaline Foods

This chapter identifies acid and alkaline foods and our body's response to them through pH testing. First, look at the food you eat and how it affects urine and saliva pH. Dr. Christopher Vasey, ND authored a book on <u>The Acid-Alkaline Diet for Optimum Health</u>.[8] He claims that creating proper pH balance in your diet assists in restoring health. Key points from his book include what he calls the truth – *"we are what we eat,"* process, and eliminate. He believes that today's pace, fast foods, the use of pesticides, preservatives, and artificial substances are complicators for our health, also, negative thinking (anger and unloving thoughts) has a strong acidifying effect on tissues, and affects our "inner light," he says. This concept will be discussed in the second Circle of Health.

How is a proper pH balance created? What is pH testing and how long does it take? According to Dr. Vasey, *there is no single method that can give a complete picture of the body's pH. There are two simple methods of urine and saliva pH testing. The first is over a two-day period. The second is over a five-day period, testing at 10 a.m. after discarding the first urine of the day, and then at 2 p.m. and bedtime. The two or five days give an average of readings over time.* Another school of thought from various resources suggests that testing of saliva and urine (excluding the first urine of the day) should occur at different times throughout the day since various times of the day, stress, foods and activities all affect pH results. The results, then, can be utilized to adjust the type of food consumption and selection of pH supplements to normalize the pH.

According to Dr. Vasey in his pamphlet, "pH Health Assessment",[9] " *'p' comes from potential. 'H' is the symbol for the element Hydrogen, so pH means potential for Hydrogen, and pH is simply a measurement of acidity and alkalinity.*" Dr. Vasey also says, "*The pH scale is 0-14 and 7 is neutral. Ideal blood pH needs to be in the range of 7.35-7.45.*" According to other sources, the stomach has a pH of 2-3, and the urine and saliva range is 6.1-6.6. Understanding what pH is, and how foods affect pH, is essential when choosing foods for a healthier lifestyle.

Dr. Vasey[8] and Robert and Shelley Young[10] listed several examples of conditions resulting from high acidity:

Allergies	*Hot flashes*
Asthma	*Insomnia*
High blood pressure	*Lack of energy/ chronic fatigue*
High blood sugar	*Inflammation of joints*
Depression	*Stiffness*
Digestive problems	*Skin problem*
Fungal problems	*Weight issues*
Headaches	*Premature aging*
Heartburn	*AIDs*

Colds/flu   *PMS*

MS   *Diabetes*

According to Dr. Vasey,[8] *toxicity leads to microform overgrowth of pathogens, yeast, fungi, and parasites that may lead to illnesses.* "*Fat is an excellent binding agent... and stores toxins in your body,*" Dr. Vasey also stated. "*Your weight problem is more complex than a simply a metabolic problem. It is really an ACID problem.*"

"*Cells have a positive electrical charge on the inside (acid),*" stated Dr. Vasey, "*and a negative electrical charge on the outside (alkaline).*"[9] "*Over 65 % of your body weight is made up of intracellular and extracellular fluid (totaling 11-16 gallons). Those fluids must remain in an alkaline pH ...,*" Dr. Vasey continued. *Our body also rids itself of 500 million cells that die and are replaced daily, the Youngs stated.*[10]

There are three things that cause acidity, according to Dr. Vasey:[8]

1. *Ingestion of acids*
2. *Creation of acids*
3. *Improper elimination of acids*

Note: "*Yeast and fungus (Y/F) produce a waste product of lactic acid, and the amount of uric acid and acetaldehyde produced by Y/F is overwhelming...*" the Youngs state.[10]

In his review of those three causes, Dr. Vasey tells us, "*Acidifying foods are those that are processed - sugar, meat, dairy, coffee, alcohol, etc. These lower the pH of the body. An overload of acids can overwhelm the body's ability to neutralize them.*[9]

"Microforms such as anaerobic bacteria, yeasts and fungi proliferate when your body becomes acidic. These pathogens and microforms also create acidifying toxins in the body, thus contributing to even further acidification.... Not all acids are the same. Some are weak and some are strong. Weak acids like citric and acetic acid," says Dr. Vasey, *"are much easier to neutralize than strong acids like uric acid."*[9]

According to Dr. Vasey, *"... low urinary pH is also an indication that you are low on alkaline mineral reserves that are used to neutralize the acids eliminated by your urine.... A low saliva pH reading also indicates mineral depletion....*

Your body will leach calcium (alkaline) directly from your bones, or magnesium (alkaline) from your muscles to correct an acidic condition. ... if left unchecked, this can lead to osteoporosis, kidney stones, tooth decay...," he confirmed.[9]

Resources may differ in the ranges for urine and saliva pH. The above authors all agree that urine and saliva need to be tested regularly, at least daily. Manufacturer's recommendations on ranges should be utilized when using their litmus paper for pH testing. Proper food selections, as well as various supplements available on the market, assist in bringing the pH back into range.

Some resources recommend using three calcium supplements to bring pH back into range. They suggest using calcium lactase to bring urine and saliva alkaline readings back into range if too alkaline, calcium hydroxide to bring urine and saliva pH into range if too acidic, and calcium gluconate to maintain a pH range of 6.1 to 6.4. If saliva is alkaline, and urine is acidic, all three calcium supplements may be taken. Those supplements are available through Nutritional Resources at www.phasesoftware.com.[11]

Another resource for further information is Dr. Carey A. Reams in his book, Choose Life or Death.[12] Dr. Reams explains that foods previously were farmed with natural fertilizer and other natural methods and those chemicals were not used. Processed foods, artificial additives and preservatives, and restaurant eating affect our pH levels more today than they did in the past.

According to the Youngs,[10] *"…protein and starch should not be eaten at the same time. Digestion is affected and bacteria cause fermentation. Bad combinations are fish and chips, chicken and rice, burger and fries. Other bad food combinations are protein with sugar and sugar with starch. An example is Americans' favorite peanut butter and jelly sandwich."*

The Youngs explain that yeast and fungus have been named as *"…major players in chronic fatigue syndrome… this syndrome may also involve damage to nerve tissue by yeast, fungus, and/ or interference with nerve transmission by toxic breakdown of neurotransmitters by acetaldehyde…. Additional neurological effects that may occur from yeast and fungus include mood swings, depression, anxiety attacks, paranoia, PMS, headaches, migraines, inability to concentrate, poor memory, confusion, dizziness, and MS-like symptoms, including slurred speech and muscular incoordination...," state the Youngs. "Microforms and their toxins contribute directly or indirectly to many symptoms of pain, infection, fatigue, diabetes, respiratory problems, tumors, cysts, allergies, lack of sex drive etc.... These are just some of the illnesses that may be caused by yeast and fungus toxins from an acid-laden diet."[10]*

According to the Youngs, once the colon is cleansed, the following "WOMAN" steps are recommended. "WOMAN" refers to water, oxygenation, minerals, alkalize, and nutritional supplements as follows:[10]

"Water – drink alkaline water, up to 128 ounces per day...."[10] Other sources recommend drinking at least half of one's body weight in ounces of water. Others suggest adding chlorine dioxide to water to increase alkalinity. Still others say to drink when thirsty.

"Oxygenation - various techniques using super hydration with oxygenated, structured water; exercise; breathing techniques; lymphatic massage therapy; alkaline baths, and castor oil wraps."[10]

"Minerals act as cofactors in the production of energy, assist in production of metabolic enzymes and utilization of vitamins, and chelate exotoxins and mycotoxins."[10] Minerals are present in the foods we eat. Since foods are picked before they are ripe, they lack certain minerals when taken to market. In mass farming, with its added pesticides and chemicals, foods lack the nutrients needed to process in the body effectively. Dr. Bill H. McAnalley[13] patented the breakthrough product, glyconutrients. This vital supplement of cellular

communication has had a major, positive, health influence when added to the daily routine. For more information, go to www.mymannapages.com/susanhallnd. Another resource explaining this concept is called Sugars that Heal.[14]

"Alkalize – alkalize with fresh green juices and a green foods diet."[10] This includes fresh, raw, dark, green, leafy foods.

"Nutritional supplements – supplementation with nano-colloidal formulations, botanicals, and other essential ingredients to bring the body back into balance."[10]

Note: Too much alkalinity can affect the kidneys. Remember, do everything in moderation to get the pH in neutral range and keep it there. The Youngs state *that parasites, yeast, and bugs do not thrive at 6.4.*[10] Once the pH in our urine and saliva is out of the 6.1-6.6 range, essential vitamins and trace minerals are lost. They include *iodine, moly, silver, germanium, selenium, copper, zinc, chromium, manganese, iron, cobalt, sulphur, chlorine, potassium, calcium, titanium, vanadium, sodium, magnesium, silica, phosphorous, hydrogen, carbon, lithium, beryllium, boron, nitrogen, oxygen, fluorine, and vitamins A, B, E, F, and K.*

There are many supplements and dietary suggestions to aid our digestive system. Some foods, *when digested, are considered an "ash."*[8] The pH of "ash" is different from the pH of food. *"For example, a lemon is acidic,"* explains Dr. Vasey, *"but once digested has a very alkalizing effect. This is because the acid in a lemon (citric acid) is a weak acid,"* he said. *"The acid converts to water and CO_2" (which is acidic) and exhaled by the* *lungs."*[9]

Good food choices, proper storage, and cooking when appropriate, play important roles in keeping our pH in balance according to the Youngs' theory.[10] Food becomes more acidic when cooked, and some foods should be totally avoided. The Youngs recommend the following dos and don'ts for a healthy lifestyle:[10]

1. *Avoid junk foods.*

2. *Avoid fruits.*

3. *Avoid pork, beef, chicken, eggs, dairy, animal food.*

4. *Avoid all microwaved foods.*

5. *Avoid all products containing baker's brewer's yeast.*

6. *Avoid dairy products.*

7. *Avoid condiments.*

8. *Avoid malt products.*

9. *Avoid edible fungi.*

10. *Avoid alcohol.*

11. *Avoid all products containing caffeine.*

12. *Avoid peanuts and peanut products.*

13. *Avoid corn and corn products.*

14. *Avoid smoking and/or chewing tobacco.*

15. *Avoid heated oils at all costs.*

16. *Eat a lot of dark green and yellow vegetables, preferably raw. But if this causes uncomfortable bloating and gas, lightly steam until the body is use to digesting these.*

17. *Limit stored grains.*

18. *The best foods are sprouts.*

19. *Carbohydrates, vegetables, legumes and unstored grains except corn are allowed.*

20. *Soy products for protein and other nutrients are recommended.*

21. *Fresh water fish is recommended.*

22. *Water is necessary for hydration.*

23. *Sweat your way to radiate health.*

24. *Take daily vitamin and mineral supplements.*

25. *Use fresh herbs and spices.*

The ratio of alkaline foods to acidic foods should be 80% alkaline to 20% acidic, or 4:1 according to the Youngs.[10] Dr. Vasey presented the following lists as examples of foods that range from acidic to alkaline: [9]

Highly alkaline foods include:

Juices from grasses (wheat germ, kamut grass, barley grass, etc.); green vegetables (cucumbers, spinach, celery, green peppers, *peas, leafy greens); watercress, cabbage, turnips, red beets, red radishes, chard, cilantro, <u>limes, fresh lemons, tomatoes,</u> egg plant, avocadoes, fresh soy beans, sprouted seeds, white beans, air-dried soy nut, sea salt, and alkaline water.*

Moderately alkaline foods include:

Asparagus, artichokes, bananas, carrots, white radishes, rutabagas, raw sweet potatoes, <u>buckwheat</u> grouts, soy flour, <u>spelt,</u> tofu, almonds (very good), brazil nuts, hazelnuts, pumpkin seeds, sunflower seeds, flax seeds, sesame seeds, cumin seeds, fennel seeds, caraway seeds, fresh herbs, cold pressed oils and stevia. <u>Garlic, ginger, and onions are naturals for anti-fungal and anti-parasitical benefits.</u>

Note: All foods underlined are highly recommended.

Mildly alkaline foods include:

Cherries, watermelons, grapefruits, fresh figs, cantaloupe, dates, plums, raspberries, blueberries, strawberries, black currants, cranberries, ripe grapes, ripe gooseberries, tangerines, mangos, oranges, papaya, apricots, peaches, pears, apples, brown rice, wild rice, grains and beans, walnuts, pecans, spelt, back-eyed peas, string beans, packaged natural vegetable broth, and bragg liquid aminos.

Highly acidic foods include:

Canned, processed and microwaved foods, all fried foods, ice cream, cottonseed oil, pudding, jams and jellies, anything hydrogenated, candy, packaged snacks, chocolate, cola and soft drinks, coffee and black tea, liquor, wine, beer.

Moderately acidic foods include:

Fish, turkey, chicken, eggs, white bread, white rice, white biscuits, shrimp, lobster, crab cakes, pastries, and pasta.

Slightly acidic foods include:

Fructose, milk sugar, turbinado sugar, margarine, corn oil, vanilla, tapioca, cashews, processed soybeans, hard cheese, peanuts, pistachios, and apple cider vinegar.

According to the Youngs,[10] it seems as though all the foods we enjoy are the ones to avoid. Remember, on rare occasions, you can eat some highly acidic foods, but not every day. Additional information on this topic is available from the Youngs in their book, <u>The pH Miracle for Weight Loss.</u>[15]

Although the Youngs do not agree with eating fruits, other natural health practitioners believe one of the best rules of thumb is to eat fruit or protein in the morning. Starches digest within four to five hours, so eating vegetables with a starch for lunch provides energy during the day. The evening meal should be full of protein for growth of our cells. Any non-starch with a protein is a good combination.

Good fats provide warmth and insulation for the body. We should eat when hungry, and eat green foods (preferably raw or steamed vegetables) before a protein. Other resources recommend fasting from solid foods and drinking clear liquids at least one day a month to cleanse the body.

In order to explore how foods and lifestyle affect pH, twelve volunteers agreed to test their pH of urine and saliva according to Dr. Vasey's program.[9]

Volunteers' pH Results

Twelve volunteers (six males, six females) whose ages ranged from 35-72 years, with varying health conditions, agreed to be pH tested for this research study. Using pH sticks, they tested their saliva and urine. There are also other products that measure pH such as litmus paper. The focus was to measure how their eating habits and other activities affected their pH.

The methods used for this urine and saliva pH testing were simple. It has been suggested that two days are necessary for properly testing the body's pH levels.[8] Other schools of thought include testing over a five-day period beginning at 10:00 a.m. (after discarding the first urine of the day), again at 2:00 p.m. and then at bedtime.[8] Whichever time frame is used, readings are to be averaged over that time period. For this study, testing was accomplished over a two-day period.

In order to self-test on a regular basis, take readings at

various times throughout the day. Rather than waiting to average results over a two to five-day period, adjust foods and supplements according to immediate results. (Don't forget to discard the first urine of the day.)

The volunteers' results fell in these general pH zones: [9]

pH 4.5 to 5.75 *-very Acidic zone*	There were 3 males in this zone.
pH 6.0 to 6.5 *is the Acidic zone*	There were 7 people in this zone.
pH 6.75-7.25 is the *Optimal zone*	Only 1 female was in this zone.
pH 7.5 – 9.0 is the *very Alkaline zone*	Only 1 female was in this zone.

Individuals were informed of their test results. In the bell curve of results, the majority fell in the optimal range for urine and saliva pH. They were provided with information about adjusting food choices to bring them within the ideal pH range. It was recommended that they change their lifestyles one day at a time, and they were reminded that it is a process and does not happen overnight. They also were advised to test their pH at various times of the day (discarding the first urine upon arising), and to adjust foods and take some type of acid-alkaline supplement. The one I recommend is called pH Buffer and is obtained from www.vaxa.com.[16]

CHAPTER III

Supplements and Organic Foods

Supplements

Dr. Alex Duarte from <u>The Untold Truth</u> series, 'Running on Empty,'[17] offers seven recommendations as follows:

Multivitamins, trace minerals, and antioxidant supplements assist in weight loss, fortify the immune system, and increase energy.

Probiotics are a good form of bacteria needed to boost your immune system and improve digestion. They are especially needed if you have a history of antibiotic use that has destroyed good bacteria.

Enzymes are needed to assist the body's digestive system. They also restore pH balance and vitamin-mineral absorption, reduce metabolic acidity and diminish the workload of the pancreas and liver, keeping blood sugar stable.

It is important to increase essential fatty acids, mainly the Omega 3s, since we get Omega 6s from our foods.

Raw fruits and vegetables feed probiotics, absorb toxins and carry cholesterol out of the body. Fiber and whole grains promote a healthy colon, regulate digestive processes, and help keep blood sugar even.

Fruit blends that serve as antioxidants protect against inflammation include wolfberry, mangosteen, concord concentrate, blueberry and red raspberry concentrates, etc.

Water is essential for organ and tissue hydration and for moving through the digestive system. It also eliminates toxins.

Weight loss is often hampered by stress, according to Dr. Duarte. Abdominal (belly) fat is the body's response to stress and its triggers, he maintains. A cortisol supplement supports our adrenals that are affected by stress. Another herbal supplement that helps with stress and weight management is licorice root. Those supplements can be obtained through Nature's Sunshine.

My Nature's Sunshine products also offer a dieter's cleanse to detoxify the colon and glands. Then, by taking their Skinny Formula (SF) for six to eight weeks, you can curb your appetite and aid in daily elimination. Those are just a few supplements that can assist a healthy lifestyle. There are many more.

Organic Foods

Be choosy about buying food. There are at least ten reasons to purchase organic foods for our meals. According to <u>The Encyclopedia of Natural Healing</u> by Seigfried Gursche and Rona Zoltan,[18] *"Organic food is grown or produced without using harmful pesticides, fungicides or chemical fertilizers. 'Certified organic' means that an independent certifying agency* has regularly inspected the farm to ensure that water and soil meet the standards for organic food."

"All foods can be produced organically, including fruits, vegetables, grains, beans, seeds, nuts, meat, and dairy products," according to Seigfried Gursche, MH, Zoltan Rona, MD, MSc."[18] Why buy organic?

Organic food tastes better. Produce is nourished by mineral-rich soil, picked with care when ready, and packed by people who are concerned with taste, quality and health. With organic food, you get more nutrition for your money. Conventional food costs somewhat less, but has much less nutritional value. Organic food is produced from soil that has been enriched with natural compost and has high levels of nutrients and trace minerals.

Conventional food has many hidden costs that are not reflected in the price, including costs for environmental clean-ups, pesticide and fertilizer regulation, and subsidies to conventional farms. The cost of care for people who develop diseases because of pesticide ingestion is not directly reflected in the price of conventional food, and neither is the cost of pollution and global climate change from the emissions of vehicles and machinery used to apply pesticides and fertilizers.

Organic food reduces your intake of harmful chemicals, and lowers your risk of getting various cancers and other illnesses. Children especially benefit from eating organic food because their immune systems are weaker than those of adults.

You support your smaller, local farmers by purchasing their organic food. These organic farmers are your neighbors and are *concerned about the health of the community. Big agri-business is more concerned with their profits than with community health.*

You protect farm workers from the cumulative, toxic effects of pesticides and chemical fertilizers by purchasing organic food.

Organic farmers help to ensure a sustainable agriculture for future generations by increasing the soil's natural vitality and mineral content.

Buying organic food protects the quality of our waters. Hundreds of tons of harmful pesticides and fertilizers are washed into our rivers, lakes and oceans every year, polluting drinking water and killing fish and wildlife.

Organic farmers help restore biodiversity because they use natural crop diversification. Conventional farmers use harmful monoculture and harsh chemicals to produce large quantities of a single crop.

Conventional farmers sometimes produce food that has been manipulated genetically, changing the essential nature of the food. Organic farmers believe the natural state of food is the best for health, and they reject genetic manipulation as dangerous and harmful.

We have discussed supplements, organic foods, and acid/alkaline foods. Next is food selections based on our blood type. We are more than halfway through our first circle of health, "...and the physical is the result."[1]

CHAPTER IV

Blood Types and Food Selections

The concept of blood types and food selections was previously touched upon. Dr. Peter J. D'Adamo[7] discusses the four blood types and how each is affected by foods. Each blood group possesses a different antigen with its own special chemical structure.

According to Dr. D'Adamo, "...*blood groups are named for their antigen structures.*"[7] *For example, blood group A has an A antigen on its red blood cell. Blood group B has a B antigen. Blood group AB has both AB antigens, and Blood group O has no true antigen. All human blood, with exceedingly rare exceptions, carries the red cell H antigen. It is primarily present in O red cells, and least present in AB cells.*

Dr. D'Adamo continues to say that *Group O has no true antigen, and produces antibodies against all the other blood groups. Group O can only receive blood from another O. Group A produces anti-B antibodies and cannot receive blood from B or AB. Group B produces anti-A antibodies and cannot receive blood from A or AB. Group AB produces no antibodies and is the "universal receiver." Group O produces no antigen for other blood groups to react to, and is the "universal donor."*

Dr. D'Adamo continues, "If you follow your Blood Type Plan carefully, you can:

Avoid many common viruses and infections.

Lose weight as your body rids itself of toxins and fats.

Fight back against life-threatening diseases such as cancer, cardiovascular disease, diabetes, and liver failure.

Avoid many of the factors that cause rapid cell deterioration, thus slowing down the aging process.

The Blood Type Plan is not a panacea...."[7]

Following are examples of each blood type and foods that are helpful and harmful. "...Beneficial is a food that acts like a medicine. Avoid is a food that acts like a poison...."[7]

Blood Type AB - Beneficial foods

Meats/Fish: *mutton, lamb, turkey, cod, grouper, mahi-mahi, ocean perch, salmon, tuna, snapper, sea trout*

Beans/Legumes: *lentils, green, navy, pinto, soy-brown, black, green-edamame*

Eggs/Dairy: *nonfat cottage cheese, farmer's cheese, feta cheese, goat cheese, ricotta cheese,*

Nuts/seeds/oils: *chestnuts, flaxseeds, walnuts, olive*

Cereals/breads/pastas/grains: *oat bran, oatmeal, puffed rice, rice* *bran, spelt, brown rice, rye, rye flour*

Vegetables/fruits: *alfalfa sprouts, broccoli, cauliflower, celery, sweet potatoes, pineapple, plums, lemons, cherries*

Spices/condiments: *garlic, horseradishes, parsley*

Juices/herbal teas: *regular coffee, decaf, green tea, red wine, ginseng, ginger, strawberry, cherry, cabbage, carrot, celery, grape, papaya, hawthorn, licorice root, milk thistle, Echinacea*

Blood Type AB - Foods to avoid

Meats/fish: *bacon, beef, buffalo, chicken, Cornish hens, duck, goose, pork of all kinds, venison, quail, bluegill, bass, sea bass, farmed-raised salmon, shrimp, striped bass, turtle*

Beans/legumes: *adzuki, black, black-eyed peas, Lima, kidney*

Eggs/dairy: *American cheese, blue cheese, brie, buttermilk, ice cream, whole milk, sherbet, parmesan, provolone*

Nuts/seeds/oils: *poppy seeds, pumpkin seeds, sesame butter, sunflower seeds, corn, cottonseed, safflower*

Cereals/breads/pastas/grains: *buckwheat, corn flakes, corn muffins, artichoke, barley flour, corn meal, soba noodles*

Vegetables/fruits: *artichokes, white and yellow corn, black olives, red, yellow and green peppers, radishes, bananas, coconuts, mangos, oranges, persimmons, pomegranates, pears, rhubarb*

Spices/condiments: *allspice, almond extract, anise, barley, malt, cayenne, cornstarch, corn syrup, ketchup, black pepper, tapioca,* *white vinegar, Worcestershire sauce*

Beverages/herbal teas: *black tea- regular and decaf, sodas, corn silk, red clover, rhubarb, orange juice, mango*

Blood Type B - Beneficial Foods

Meats/fish: *mutton, lamb, rabbit, cod, grouper, mahi-mahi, ocean perch, salmon, tuna, sardines, sea trout, halibut, pike, sole*

Beans/legumes: *kidney, Lima, navy, black and brown soybeans, green edamame*

Eggs/dairy: *cottage cheese, farmer's cheese, feta cheese, goat cheese, low-fat mozzarella cheese, low-fat ricotta cheese, goat's milk, skim or 2 percent milk, yogurt*

Nuts/oils: *macadamia, olive*

Cereals/breads/pastas/grains: *millet, oat bran, oatmeal, puffed millet, puffed rice, rice bran, spelt, brown rice bread, rice cakes, rice pasta, spelt pasta*

Vegetables/fruits: *Florida avocados, beets, broccoli, Brussels sprouts, white carrots, egg plant, parsley, parsnips, potatoes, yams, bananas, cranberries, kiwi, papaya, pineapples*

Spices/ condiments: *Cayenne pepper, curry, ginger, horseradish, parsley*

Blood Type B - Foods to avoid

Meat/fish: *chicken, Cornish hens, duck, goose, all kinds of pork, quail, crab, lobster, farm-raised salmon, sea bass, shrimp, snail, turtle, yellowtail*

Beans/legumes: *adzuki, black, black-eyed peas, garbanzo, lentils, green, pinto*

Eggs/dairy: *American cheese, blue cheese, ice cream, string cheese*

Nuts/seeds/oils: *cashews, filberts, peanuts, peanut butter, pine, pistachio, poppy seeds, pumpkin seeds, sesame butter, sesame seeds, sunflower butter, canola, corn, cottonseed, peanut, safflower, sesame, sunflower*

Cereals/breads/pastas/grains: *barley, buckwheat, corn flakes, cream of wheat, kamut, rye, seven grain, shredded wheat, wheat bran, corn muffins, rye crisp, rye bread, ryvita, wheat bagels, wheat-bran muffins, whole wheat, barley flour, buckwheat, cornmeal, wheat, gluten flour, rye, whole wheat flour, wild rice.*

Vegetables/fruits: *yellow and white corn, black, Greek, green, and Spanish olives, pumpkin, radishes, tomatoes, coconut, persimmons, pomegranates, rhubarb, pears*

Spices/condiments: *allspice, almond extract, barley malt, cinnamon, cornstarch, corn syrup, plain gelatin, ketchup, black and white ground pepper, tapioca*

Beverages/herbal teas: *tomatoes, aloe, corn silk, goldenseal, hops, linden, rhubarb, distilled liquor, sodas*

Blood Type A - Beneficial foods

Meats/fish: *no meats, carp, cod, ocean salmon, rainbow trout, snapper, sardines, sea trout, perch, white fish, yellow perch*

Beans/legumes: *adzuki, black peas, green, pinto, black and brown* soy, green edamame

Eggs/dairy: soy cheese, soy milk

Nuts/seeds/oils: flaxseed, organic peanut butter, pumpkin seeds, redskin peanuts, unsalted, linseed, olive

Cereals/breads/pastas/grains: kasha, millet bread, oat, rye, rice cakes, oat flour, rice pasta, soba noodles, spelt noodles

Vegetables/fruits: broccoli, carrots, chicory, horseradishes, parsley, parsnips, pumpkin, romaine lettuce, spinach, tofu, turnips, apricots, blackberries, blueberries, cherries, cranberries, dried and fresh figs, grapefruit, lemons, pineapple, plums, red, prunes, raisins

Spices/condiments: barley, malt, molasses, garlic, ginger, mustard, soy sauce

Beverages/herbal teas: regular and decaf coffee, green tea, red wine, water, alfalfa, burdock, chamomile, Echinacea, ginger, ginseng, hawthorn, milk thistle, rose hips, St. John's wort, apricots, blackberries, carrot, celery, grapefruit, pineapple prune, water, and lemons

Blood Type A - Foods to avoid

Meats/fish: beef, buffalo, duck, goose, heart, lamb, liver, pheasant, all pork, rabbit, veal, venison, quail, bluefish, sea bass, halibut, herring, lobster, shrimp, mussels, turtle, striped bass

Beans/Legumes: copper, kidney, Lima, navy, red

Eggs/dairy: American cheese, blue cheese, brie, buttermilk, cheddar, Colby, cottage cheese, cream cheese, ice cream, skim and 2% milk, parmesan, provolone, sherbet, nonfat sour cream, Swiss, whey

Nuts/seeds: Brazil, cashews, pistachio, corn, cottonseed, peanut, safflower, sesame

Cereals/ breads/pastas/grains: cream of wheat, granola, grape nuts, shredded wheat, wheat germ, wheat bran, seven grain, English muffins, high-protein bread, pumpernickel, wheat bran muffins, wheat matzos, whole wheat bread, semolina pasta, spinach pasta, white/whole wheat flour

Vegetables/fruits: red and white cabbage; eggplant; mushrooms; black, Greek, and Spanish olives; red, yellow, and green peppers; white, red, and sweet potatoes; tomatoes; yams; bananas; coconuts; mangos; melons; cantaloupe; honeydew; oranges; papaya; rhubarb; tangerines

Spices/condiments: capers, ketchup, mayonnaise, black pepper, red pepper flakes, peppercorn, relish-all kinds, apple cider, balsamic, red and white vinegar, wintergreen, Worcestershire sauce

Beverages/herbal teas: beer, liquor, seltzer water, sodas, orange, papaya, tomato, regular and decaf black tea

Blood type O - Beneficial foods

Meats/fish: Beef, ground beef, buffalo, lamb, liver, mutton, veal, venison, cod, halibut, fresh herring, mackerel, pike, rainbow trout, red snapper, salmon, sardines, sole, swordfish, white perch, white fish, yellow tail perch

Beans/legumes: adzuki, black-eyed peas, pinto beans

Eggs/dairy: nonfat mozzarella cheese, nonfat sour cream, Body Genetics protein shakes

Nuts/seeds/oils: flaxseed, macadamia nuts, pumpkin seeds, walnuts, linseed flaxseed, olive oils

Cereals/breads/pastas/grains: no cereal, essence bread, Ezekiel bread, no pastas/grains

Vegetables/fruits: domestic and Florida artichokes, beet leaves, broccoli, collard greens, dandelion, kale, red peppers, romaine lettuce, plums, sweet potatoes, pumpkin, seaweed, spinach, Swiss chard, turnips, dried and fresh figs

Spices/condiments: carob, cayenne, pepper, curry, garlic, horseradish, kelp, parsley, Tabasco, turmeric

Juices/herbal teas: green tea, seltzer water, soda water, distilled water, cayenne, ginger, linden, milk thistle, mulberry, parsley, peppermint, slippery elm, black cherry, pineapple, prune

Blood type O - Foods to avoid

Meats/fish: goose, all pork, catfish, caviar, conch, pickled herring, smoked salmon, octopus

Legumes/beans: copper, kidney, navy, tamarind, green lentils, red

Nuts/seeds/oils: brazil nuts, cashews, litchi, peanuts, peanut butter, pistachios, poppy seeds, corn, cottonseed, peanut, safflower

Cereals/breads/pastas/grains: *corn flakes, cream of wheat, grape nuts, oat bran, oatmeal, shredded wheat, wheat bran, wheat germ, corn muffins, English muffins, high protein bread, multi-grain bread, oat bran muffins, pumpernickel bread, cornmeal, couscous flour, gluten flour, graham flour, oat flour, semolina, spinach pasta, soba noodles, white flour, whole wheat flour, seven grain bread, wheat bagels, wheat bran muffins, wheat matzos, whole wheat bread*

Eggs/dairy: *American cheese, blue cheese, buttermilk, cheddar, Colby, cottage cheese, ice cream, edam, kefir, 2% and skim milk, Monterey jack cheese, muenster, parmesan cheese, provolone, all types yogurt, string cheese, Swiss, whey*

Vegetables/fruits: *California avocados; cabbage; cauliflower; white corn; eggplant; domestic mushrooms; black, green, and Spanish olives; red potatoes; blackberries; cantaloupe; coconut; honeydew melon; oranges; rhubarb; tangerines*

Spices/condiments: *cinnamon, cornstarch, corn syrup, nutmeg, black, white and red pepper, ketchup, dill, kosher and sweet pickles, sucrose, relish*

Beverages/herbal teas: *coffee, distilled liquor, sodas, regular and decaf black tea, apple cider, cabbage, orange*

As you begin to look at your blood type, you can see those foods to avoid are also high in acidity. The next Chapter addresses food combinations that are yet another component for a healthy lifestyle.

CHAPTER V

Proper Food Combinations

The digestion of food is easier if foods are combined properly. The digestive system is a constant site of chemical activity, with different chemicals needed to digest each food. For example, starches require an alkaline digestive medium that is produced in the mouth by the digestive enzyme ptyalin. Proteins require an acid medium called hydrochloric acid. Acids and alkalines neutralize themselves. So, eating a protein and a starch simultaneously neutralizes and stops digestion. We derive no food value from undigested foods. If food is not digested, it rots, turns into alcohol and poisons, and leaves the stomach in a mess. Belching and gas can be symptoms of indigestion, and can cause sickness and internal poisoning.

Each enzyme, according to Lee DuBelle,[19] *has its own action, and it acts on one specific food type. Enzymes that act on protein do not act on sugars. If enzymes are heated, they are destroyed in our foods. This is why raw vegetables contain more nutrition. There is a sequence and process that stimulates each enzyme to work in the body to convert our food for nutrition. Our overall health is affected by the combination of foods and how long they take to digest throughout the day.*

There are others who have also recognized the effects of food combinations, such as Wayne Pickering, a living activist. He developed a chart of seven rules for combining food.[20]

Do not combine protein and starches. The only exception is avocados. They combine well with all starchy vegetables and grains. Legumes also combine fairly well with grains. Remember: hamburger on bread is a protein and starch combination, and it neutralizes the digestive system and can rot there.

Do not combine fruits with starches. Fruits do not require much time in the digestive system and should be eaten alone. Starches require more digestive time. Raisins in bread and cereal, and bananas in bread are bad combinations.

Do not combine fruits with proteins. Fruits are directly absorbed into the intestines. Proteins require much more time to digest. If other food remains in the stomach while waiting for protein to digest, it can rot.

Do not combine fruits with vegetables. Fruits are cleansers and vegetables are builders. Remember, a house cannot be built while cleaning it. Tomatoes are the only exception. Tomatoes can be combined with lettuce, celery, okra, cucumbers, eggplants, bell pepper, and summer squash.

Eat melons by themselves. They require little digestive time at all. If combined with other foods and held in the stomach, melons will rot. They are to be eaten alone with no exceptions.

Do not combine acid fruits with sweet fruits. Examples of this are bananas and grapefruit, oranges and raisins, tangerines and prunes. There is no exception to this.

Do not eat desserts. If you eat desserts with fruits, your digestive system is affected. Bacteria processes food into alcohol and vinegars, and no digestion occurs. The releasing of gas from the digestive system into the bowels is normal. But it's not natural to have foul-smelling gas.

The types and combinations of food we eat and their acidity or alkalinity affect our health. Our blood type is a factor in our food selection, as well as our risks for illnesses. We can learn, however, how to eat healthy.

Following these ten rules to healthy eating will guide your selection of foods:[20]

Combine foods properly.

Do not mix more than four to six fruits or vegetables at a meal.

Do not drink liquids with meals. Drink 30 minutes before, and one hour after a meal.

Never eat fried, processed, refined, enriched, canned or boxed foods.

Eat in moderation.

Chew your food. Your stomach has no teeth.

Allow at least four hours between meals, and don't eat later than four hours prior to bedtime. If you eat late at night, before going to bed, the digestive system works all night to digest food. This is why people are tired in the morning.

Eat fruits and vegetables only when ripe, when in season, according to the types of seeds it contains such as core or citrus, and when grown as close to your environment as possible. For example, Eskimos do not eat pineapple and watermelon.

Never eat anything too hot or too cold. Food should be at room temperature. Inside your stomach is 104 degrees, so if the item is too cold, it will affect the temperature and prolongs the digestive process. If food is too hot, it passes through the mouth too quickly, and therefore does not signal digestion to begin.

Always eat juicy foods before concentrated foods.

Other theories on food combinations come from the Encyclopedia of Natural Healing. [18]

Separate proteins and carbohydrates. Proteins include cheese, coconut, eggs, fish, fowl, meat, milk, nuts, olives, soybean seeds, yogurt. Carbohydrates include beans, breads, cereals, grains, lentils, potatoes, pumpkin, split peas, squash, etc.

Eat only one concentrated protein at each meal. Do not mix with fats, and oils.

Treat juices (fruits or vegetables) as whole foods.

Drink milk alone, or not at all.

Avoid desserts.

Cold foods (including liquids) inhibit digestion.

Eat fruits alone as a fruit meal.

Fruits should not be eaten between meals while other food is digesting in the stomach.

Do not eat sweet fruits and acid fruits together.

Melons are best eaten alone, but can be mixed with acid and sub acid fruits.

Acid fruits *include blackberries, grapefruit, lemons or limes, oranges, pineapple, plums (sour), pomegranate, raspberries, sour apple, strawberries.*

Sub acid fruits *include apples, apricots, blueberries, cherries, kiwi, mangos, papaya, peaches, pears, sweet plums.*

Sweet fruits *are bananas, dates, currants, figs, dried fruit, grapes, papaya, persimmons, prunes, raisins.*

Melon fruits include cantaloupe, casaba, crenshaw, honeydew, papaya melon, persian melon, muskmelon, watermelon.

Non-starchy vegetables are asparagus, beet greens, broccoli, brussels sprouts, cabbage, celery, chard, chicory, collards, cucumber, dandelion, eggplant, endive, escarole, garlic, green beans, kale, kohlrabi, leeks, lettuce, onions, parsley, radishes, scallions, spinach, sprouts, squash, sweet peppers, Swiss chard, tomatoes, turnips, watercress, zucchini.

Mild starch vegetables include artichokes, corn, cauliflower, peas, and beets.

In general, to make digestion easier and more efficient, follow these guidelines for proper food combinations. Remember, proteins require an acidic environment for digestion, while carbohydrates (starches, sugars, and fruits) require an alkaline medium. Fruits remain in the stomach for only 20-45 minutes, and should be eaten separately.

Gusche and Zoltan's recommendations include:[18]

Do not combine fats with protein.

Acid fruits and sub acid fruits may be combined, and sub acid fruits and sweet fruits may be combined.

Melons should be eaten alone.

Avoid combining two or more types of protein at one meal.

Non- starchy vegetables may be combined with starches or proteins.

In summary, proper food combinations enhance energy levels and promote health and vitality. Food that does not digest will ferment in the stomach and cause gas, stomach discomfort, and other digestive disturbances.

Regarding healthy sweeteners, Gursche and Zoltan *also state that there are several natural, unrefined sweeteners to choose from for the occasional sweet dish - organic maple syrup, powdered dates, unpasteurized honey, raw sugar cane, malt extract, fresh fruits, brown rice syrup, dried fruits and fruit juices.*[18]

In conclusion, Gursche and Zoltan *suggest that all meals should include at least 50-60% whole grains, 25-30% vegetables, 10% beans, and at least one to two bowls of soup per day. Sea vegetables such as kelp and seaweed contain nutrients, and should be used sparingly in soup. Sea salt, tamari soy sauce, or unrefined sesame oil may be used. Fish or seafood may be served several times a week, but all other animal foods should be avoided. Nuts, seeds and fruits are good snacks a few times per week, especially while in season.*[18]

Rice syrup, barley malt, and apple juice may be used to sweeten cakes, pies, or cookies and may be eaten several times a week. Avoid molasses, corn syrup, pasteurized honey, and all refined sugars. Organic maple syrup can be used sparingly. Beverages should be clear, pure spring, or well water. Bancha twig or roasted grain tea may be served at meals.[18] This contradicts other authors' opinions about no liquids at meals.

Remember that our bodies need more food that breaks down into alkaline elements since our body tissues and blood are slightly alkaline. Fresh fruits and vegetables are the most alkaline forming foods, and millet, buckwheat, corn, almonds and all sprouted seeds are more alkaline. Whole grains are slightly acidic, and the most acid-producing foods are milk products, meats, and refined flour and sugar products.

Vegetarians need extra protein and amino acid supplements.

Dentists have found white patches on patients' gums due to a shortage of those supplements.

In summary, general tips for building your health are:

Take deep breaths often. Good oxygenation is one of the keys to a healthy life and is a good stimulant for your organs and glands.

Drink lots of water, preferably distilled or alkaline. Some of the best, pure water is the juice from fruits and vegetables, purified water, or steamed, distilled water.

Get a lot of sunshine. It is the greatest promoter of digestion, feeling healthy, fertility and is nature's nerve tonic.

Be aware of nutrition and food combinations.

Engage in a fun, sweaty activity, such as walking one hour briskly every day. Use your muscles or lose them.

Take care of your inner light. Your thoughts should be positive.

Spiritual health is the key to peace and harmony. Forgive yourself and others and be a good and giving neighbor.

Keep a balanced urine and saliva pH.

Eat essential fatty acids that contain omega 3s.

Take plant enzyme supplements to aid digestion.

Eliminate waste from your body. This takes place through sweating, respiration, urination, and bowel movements (preferably within 18-24 hours of eating).

REST. It is vital!

Additional tips from Wayne Pickering[20] on foods to avoid that destroy health include:

Avoid salt, especially MSG. *The best natural source is in minerals from fruits and vegetables. Salt waterlogs tissue, robs calcium from the body, poisons the heart, irritates the nervous system ... and is the leading cause of high blood pressure.*

Avoid refined sugar. Sugar is the leading cause of stress and increases blood sugar. It causes insulin overproduction and insulin resistance, depletes B vitamins, and decreases calcium from hair, blood, bones, teeth, etc. Sugar is very toxic to the body. It contributes to the development of high cholesterol, atherosclerosis, and an over stimulation of alkaline juices. Sugar interferes with the absorption of protein, calcium and other minerals; retards intestinal growth of good bacteria; is a major contributor to diabetes; and causes fatigue – a downer, not an energizer. It also causes mental illness and memory loss.

Avoid enriched flours. Do not use white or bleached foods.

Avoid hydrogenated oils. Only use safflower, sesame, olive, soy, corn, avocado, walnut, peanut, sunflower seed, almond or apricot oil.

Milk products should also be avoided, including ice cream. Three products suggested for use are soy, seed and nut milks – including coconut – as well as mothers' breast milk. Milk causes headaches, mucous and flu. Pasteurized milk keeps bad milk in a saleable condition. Human milk develops the brain first, while cow's milk develops bones first. Milk can cause arteriosclerosis, increased blood cholesterol, pyorrhea, obesity, bad digestion from coating the stomach, abnormal calcium deposits, and a variety of allergies.

NOTE: *Avoid most condiments such as ketchup, mustard, and Worcestershire sauce, processed foods as already discussed, most meats, and day-old vegetables, premixed salads, or warmed-over potatoes.*

The last component of our first inner circle is exercise. Exercise, as well as food selections and combinations, affect *"...the physical is the result."[1]*

There is one more important aspect besides food combinations that assist the digestive process. Our digestive sytem benefits from plant enzymes. Plant enzymes can be found in a product called Juice Plus. Juice plus is the most thoroughly researched brand name nutritional product on the market today. We are suppose to eat 7 - 13 servings of fresh fruits and vegatables every day. Due to our busy lifestyles, most of us simply can't and don't. Numerous clinical studies conducted in leading universities and hospitals by investigatiors in the United States, England, Australia, Austria, Italy, and Japan show that Juice Plus :

* Delivers key antioxidants and other phytonutrients that are absorbed by the body

* Reduces oxidative stress

* Helps support a healthy immune system and protect DNA

* Postivley impacts several important indicators of cardiovascular wellness

Juice plus is made from fresh, high quality fruits and vegetables, and is carefully tested to ensure that no pesticides or other contaminants affect the natural purity of the product. These fruits and vegatables are juiced, and the juices are then concetrated into powders using a proprietary, low-tempature process. High tempatures can destroy the nutritional value of fruits and vegatables that are overcooked. Juice Plus also contains some fiber, is glutten free, fructose free and antibacterial for recovering cancer patients. The whole food based nutrition of Juice Plus + is available for less than 1.50 per day and is less than a daily cup of gourmet coffee.

The orchard blend capsule has: apple, orange, pineapple, cranberry, papaya, peach and acerola cherry. The garden blend has: carrot, parsley, beet, kale, broccoli, cabbage, spinach, tomato, oat bran, brown rice bran. As mentioned before, do your homework and research. Stop purchasing the less effective vitamins and supplemental vitamins and utilize these 2 capsules and begin a cost savings while enjoying living a healthier lifestyle. For more information go to drsusan@juiceplus.com and read the published research.

CHAPTER VI

Physical Exercise

Another important factor besides selecting and combining foods correctly is physical activity. Rest, as well as exercise, is necessary for repairing bodies.

As you are aware, seeing a physician for prevention and care and avoiding obesity are important. Walt Larimore, MD,[21] *explains that exercising at least three hours per week aids in maintaining ideal body weight, improves overall health, and reduces the risk of medical problems including diabetes, heart disease and osteoporosis.* According to Center for Disease Control, exercise *at least thirty minutes, five days a week.*[22]

Michael Murray, ND, and Dr. Joseph Pizzorno, ND, offer seven steps to exercise.[23]

Recognize the importance of physical exercise.

Consult your physician.

Select an activity you enjoy.

Monitor exercise intensity.

Do it often.

Make it fun.

Stay motivated.

Dr. Larimore's point is, *"Get started. Do not delay. Pick a form (or forms) of exercise that is enjoyable, or at least do something else enjoyable during exercise such as listening to music or books on tape."* Dr. Larimore continues, *"Exercise with a partner or a group…. Be sure to consult your doctor when deciding on what level and type of exercise would be best for you…. "*

"Physical health is also assured by proper dental health, eliminating smoking and drinking of alcohol, maintaining a lifelong, monogamous, marital relationship, using automobile safety devices, and installing and maintaining smoke and carbon dioxide detectors," according to Dr. Larimore. Those areas are not addressed here in detail, but all work together in maintaining optimal health.

Another good resource on exercising is the book <u>Fitness for Dummies</u>.[24] It discusses the same concept of *"use it, or lose it."* This book lists the keys to fitness success.

Set specific goals.

Get your fitness tested.

Dress the part.

Keep a daily exercise diary.

Pace yourself.

Work out with a buddy or join a club.

Educate yourself.

The book also discusses money matters when selecting a gym. *It recommends being aware of hidden costs; not being afraid to bargain; steering clear of long-term memberships, and asking about the club's cancellation policies.*

Tips for buying fitness products are also addressed in this book. The author warns about being taken in by the infomercial audience or "real people" offering testimonials, being swayed by seemingly scientific terminology like zero-carb dieting and thermogenic fat burners, celebrity or "expert" endorsements and adds, do not be awed by the fact that a product was awarded a U.S. patent, and to beware of the term "proven."[24]

According to the book, there are ways to judge fitness news reports, too. *Look for context, consider the source, do not assume cause and effect, look at the number of subjects, and do not make too much of animal studies.*[24]

Common fitness myths include the following:[24]

Myth: *You must exercise for 30 consecutive minutes.*

Reality: *Ten- minute sessions burn just as many calories and provide the same health benefits.*

Myth: *Lifting weights will turn you into a World Wrestling Federation contender.*

Reality: *Unless you spend hours lifting heavy weights, this is not true.*

Myth: *If you stop exercising, your muscles turn to fat.*

Reality: *Not true. Muscles will shrink. Fat and muscle are two different entities, and cannot turn into each other.*

Myth: *By focusing on abdominal exercises, you can lose that beer gut.*

Reality:You can't selectively zap fat off a particular part of the body. To lose a beer gut, you need to lose weight, exercise, and cut down on the beer.

Myth: Exercising during pregnancy increases the rate of miscarriage or birth defects.

Reality: With a doctor's approval, prenatal exercise is very healthy for you and your body. In fact, exercise makes labor and delivery easier, as is returning to your pre- pregnancy weight.

The first six chapters conclude the first circle of health and summarize our food choices, pH, supplements, food combinations, food selections based on blood types, acid/ alkaline choices, and exercise. All of those factors contribute to "...*and the physical is the result.*"[1]

"Mind is the Builder..." [1]
~Edgar Cayce

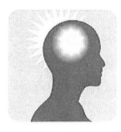

PART TWO

SECOND CIRCLE OF HEALTH

Mental Health: Inner Light and Emotions

This chapter introduces concepts that affect mental health and, ultimately, your physical well-being. The mind is very powerful and does affect physical health. The following resources will aid in self-evaluation and decision-making and will allow exploration of those ideas.

CHAPTER VII

The Inner Light, Your Subconscious Mind

Many naturopathic authors talk about our two worst mental
enemies - guilt and fear. Our patterns of living, what we
eat, our daily activities, and the way we think and feel affect
our mind, body, and emotions. All the correct eating and
exercise will not help if we are not happy and at peace and
in harmony with those around us. The mind and body
are inseparable. Don't worry about what other people
are thinking or about your position in life. Remember that
peace and happiness are the goals and are internal. It is not
what life throws at us, it is how we handle it, as my parents
always said.

According to Wayne Pickering, some key concepts for
keeping that inner light burning and to achieve emotional
health are:[20]

Stay busy.

*Practice smiling and mean it. It takes 75 muscles to frown and 15
to smile.*

Be a friend of man.

Silence is golden. Never argue - just say "yes." Questions are answered in the soul, not by arguments.

Think good, positive thoughts. Inner light is important, and affects the body's response to life. Being positive creates a brighter light.

Live one day at a time.

Know yourself, and be yourself.

Show sincere appreciation for others and applaud.

Be the best at what you do.

Write things down.

Savor simple pleasures.

Keep an open mind.

Do not procrastinate.

Write down 50 things that you're grateful for.

Save 10% of your money and give it away to others.

Janet Hranicky, PhD, researched mind/body medicine. In the book <u>Alternative Medicine, the Definitive Guide</u>,[25] Dr. Hranicky states that *"...thoughts and emotions have a direct impact on one's energy level and on the bioenergy field that surrounds the body. People who are beset with poverty, long-term loneliness, or the loss of a loved one are far more vulnerable to illness and death,"* she says. *"Mood, attitude and belief can affect virtually every chronic illness. Fear and cynicism, as well as a sense of hopelessness and helplessness, can have a detrimental effect on health. Good humor, courage, a sense of control, and hopefulness can all benefit our health. Optimists are less likely to become ill, but if they do, they tend to live longer and suffer less. How one thinks may be a predictor of well being and future health."*

Dr. Hranicky also says that *"...energy is paramount. It takes energy for the body to heal. Excitement and passion produce high energy, whereas pain and hopelessness create low energy and fear. Anxiety creates chaotic patterns. In mind/body medicine, emotions are viewed as indicators of one's state of consciousness, and have everything to do with the body's bioenergy field."*

Numerous research studies show that our conscious mind can influence our body's responses. Although our life experiences and our genes also affect our bodies, the mind has the most powerful influence.

Dr. Hranicky encourages self-examination about how healthy your beliefs and thoughts are with the following questions:[28]

Are your thoughts based on facts?

Do your thoughts /beliefs help to protect your life and health?

Do your thoughts/beliefs help you reach your short and long-term goals?

Do your thoughts/beliefs help you avoid your most undesirable conflict?

Do your thoughts/beliefs make you feel the way you want to feel?

"If you answered NO to any three of these questions, the belief or thought is considered unhealthy and needs to be changed," according to Dr. Hranicky.

Studies have shown that supportive social relationships, friends, extended family, marital ties, and group membership have a positive effect on health and the healing process.

According to Eunice Ingham,[26] *"The state of mind affects digestion more than almost any other bodily ailment. Constipation is often a state of mind."* Studies published by Dr. Boris Kaplan indicated, *"…that financial troubles might cause stomach disorders which become ulcers. The worries affect digestion, and digestive troubles increase the worry."*

"There is not an organ in the body that is not affected by the mind. Every thought we think," Dr. Kaplan continues, *"either has a constructive or destructive effect on the chemical content of our blood stream."* He says that when thoughts of fear, worry, anxiety or grief overcome us, the acidity of our bloodstream increases. Worry is a magnified form *of fear, an idea by which we torment ourselves, a fixation of attention,* he concludes.

Eunice Ingham explains, *"…our health is controlled by fixed ideas."* She continues to say, *"…most of our nervous derangements are brought about by uncontrolled emotions. A suggestion can sometimes prove a power to determine a destiny."*[26] She further asks *if we are letting fearful thoughts kill our bodies'* cells. *She notes how epidemics have been made worse by increased fear. All of our cells respond to the power of suggestion,* she claims.

Eunice Ingham further explains *that it is a fact that the body is affected by the mind! Every flitting change of the mind causes a chemical change in the body. Circulation follows attention,* she states. *The center of every cell in the body is composed of the same grey matter as the brain. Every time we think a thought, we use up energy,* she notes. Then why continue to poison the system and waste energies by harboring destructive thoughts of fear, worry, envy, and jealousy? *We cannot change natural law, she continues. But, the more truth learned the about the laws of nature that rule and govern health, which are also God's laws, the quicker systems are freed from destructive agents and the depletion of body cells.*[26]

"*Our mind can change a demand. Our ideals can be changed by a new thought,*" according to Eunice Ingham. She also states that there are authorities that say "*...cancer is caused by long continuous nerve retention. Gall bladder trouble may be brought on by anxiety. Constipation may be instigated by obstinacy, and some forms of rheumatism may be a state of the unconscious unwillingness to face the problems of life.*"[26] It may or not be true, but it is something to consider. "*There is no doubt that one's predominant mental impression is what governs the mind and the functioning of every part of one's being - even to the tiniest cell,*" she adds.

Ingham continues to explain that "*...emotions constitute the main spring of life, the driving force for good or ill effects. We* *cannot separate the power of emotions from that of mind and thought. This explains why the number of victims suffering from stomach ulcers has been known to go up or down with stock market quotations. This tells the story of some improper glandular balance, undoubtedly caused by excessive nervous tension."*[26]

According to Ingham, *"The power of thought can make us live or die. Yes, the power of our thoughts can make us live a happy and healthy life, or fill our body with poison, resulting in pain and disease.... Fear is a poison that can affect every part of the human organism." Regrets or worry also affect the body,* she continues." *Worry is derived from a Saxon word that means to choke."* Worry chokes off the body's normal blood supply to various parts of the body, Ingham says. Fear and worry create tension and the inability to relax. *"Our only limitation in the achievements of tomorrow will be our fears of today,"* according to Ingham. She warns against generating *"more indignation than you have the capacity to control.... Anger produces more poison than fear."*[26]

It is evident that the mind does affect the body. So, what phrases, thoughts and words affect one's subconscious mind, ultimately affecting the body's responses?

According to Wayne Pickering,[20] our body responds:

100% by saying, "I did."

90% by saying, "I will."

80% response with, "I can."

70% with the words, "I think I can."

60% by the words, "I might."

50% by the words, "I think I might."

40% with the words, "What is it?"

30% with the words, "I wish I could."

20% with the words, "I don't know how."

10% with the words, "I can't."

0% with words such as, "I won't."

Which of Pickering's phrases do you use most when facing a tough decision?

Dr. Joseph Murphy, PhD, is another author who agrees with Eunice Ingham and Wayne Pickering about the power of words and how they feed our subconscious minds. He discusses this concept in his book, The Power of Your Subconscious Mind.[27] He notes that using your imagination gives you the power to actually accomplish things.

Many cultures have been studied on how they respond to life. It has been found that those who live life in a positive manner live longer, according to Dr. Walt Larimore.[21] He studied the characteristics of non-Americans centenarians, and discovered:

They exercise regularly and consistently.

They avoid highly processed foods. In fact, none of their food is highly processed, as are many of our junk and fast foods....

They eat a nutritious diet. They don't overeat, and their diet is high in fiber, whole grains, nuts, and "good" fats....low in calories, salt, saturated fats, and refined sugars.

They drink lots of water...usually from wells or mountain streams and it contains a high mineral content.

They consume plenty of fresh fruits and vegetables.

They avoid loneliness. Relationships within their communities with neighbors, family and friends are vital.

They practice and enjoy regular sex – usually with their spouse, who is their longtime partner in a mutually monogamous relationship, even after the age of one hundred.

They live with, and depend on, their extended families, who offer cradle-to-grave security and support. The concept of nursing homes is unheard of, and would not be tolerated.

They seldom use alcohol or tobacco products.

They intensely respect their elders.

They lead active, fruitful lives well into their second century.

They emphasize relationships and harmony over the pursuit of wealth or success.

Those concepts were found to be significant to the centenarians' mental heath. They did not compare themselves to others because it creates inferiority complexes and serves no purpose. According to Larimore they mastered viewing oneself with a positive image as God saw them.[21]

Another concept, forgiveness of ourselves and others, has a direct impact on our mental health. Some tips on forgiveness, according to Dr. Walt Larimore, 10 Essentials of Highly Healthy People,[21] are:

F is forgiving others, starting with yourself. Look for the good in the bad.

O is for organizing one's thoughts in writing. Journaling is a powerful tool for recognizing and releasing pain.

R is for reviewing experiences. Make an effort to feel another person's feelings, seeking to figure out and understand motivation, identifying with the pressures that may have driven that person to cause hurt or pain. Being forgiven by God and others gives emotional freedom, and helps one extend forgiveness to others.

G is giving the boot to anger and regret. Confession is good for health. Asking God and others we have wronged for forgiveness is a form of healing, and releases anger and regrets.

I is for investing in removing resentment. Highly healthy people are not blamers. They take responsibility for their own thoughts and actions. They apologize and accept punishment and make restitution. They work at banishing grudges and resentment, and make a conscious choice to forgive.

V is for victory that comes from forgiving others. "To err is human, to forgive is divine." Forgiveness is not forgetting the hurt, but it is treating the person who harmed you as though the hurt did not happen. It's an act of will to do this.

I is for increasing your gratitude for past pain. Rejoice in suffering, because suffering produces perseverance. Perseverance produces character, character produces hope, and hope does not disappoint.

N *is for navigating to inner peace. This inner peace can be realized with therapies such as yoga, music therapy, aromatherapy, a hot bath, a walk in a peaceful setting, deep breathing, etc. The most important peace is the one with our Creator 'which transcends all understanding. He will guard your hearts and your minds.'*

G *is for giving comfort to others. By giving comfort, we receive comfort.*

Dispensing mercy and grace makes for highly healthy people.

This concludes the second inner circle – *"Mind is the builder…"*[1]. Next, we will explore spirituality.

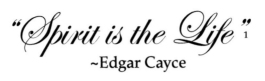

"Spirit is the Life" [1]
~Edgar Cayce

PART THREE

THIRD CIRCLE OF HEALTH

Spiritual Health: Values and Beliefs

This chapter will explore various authors' concepts on spirituality. There is no one set of spiritual guidelines. This is a personal determination for each person. For the purpose of this book, I shall utilize areas most familiar to me. Below are concepts about spirituality and the values and beliefs that affect the choices we ultimately make about our life and health.

CHAPTER VIII

Spiritual Growth and Holiness

In his book, <u>10 Essentials of Highly Healthy People</u>, Walter Larimore, MD,[21] discusses our relationship with God. He said this relationship promotes wellness and welfare of self and others, and includes the beliefs and values by which individuals live. The results are the *"... visible, spiritual fruit of love, joy, peace, patience, kindness, goodness, faithfulness, gentleness and self-control."*

Dr. Larimore's book includes medical studies that point to physical differences between those who both prayed and attended regular religious services. *"The vast majority of these studies demonstrated that a patient's religious and spiritual beliefs can be clinically beneficial and play an important in both coping with and recovering from illness,"* according to Dr. Larimore. He also states that a few of the many positive findings include:

Longer life

Lowered blood pressure

Improved surgical outcomes

Shorter hospital stays,

Improved mental health

Overall well-being.

> *"True Spirituality,"* Larimore said, *"is the path to spiritual wholeness. For most of us it's a lifelong pursuit."*[21]

There are other spiritual resources that assist in spiritual growth, and ultimately affect our health. In Joel Osteen's book, <u>Your Best life Now</u>,[28] he enumerates seven basic concepts for enhancing spiritual growth.

Enlarge your vision.

Develop a healthy self-image.

Discover the power of your thoughts and words.

Let go of the past.

Find strength through adversity.

Live to give.

Choose to be happy.

In his book, <u>Become a Better You</u>,[29] Joel Osteen proposes that it is important to do the following:

Keep pressing forward.

Be positive toward yourself.

Develop better relationships.

Form better habits.

Embrace the place where you are.

Develop your inner life.

Stay passionate about life.

Those concepts are detailed in Osteen's two books, and define how *"spirit is the life."*[1]

Other authors who have valuable advice that can advance our spiritual life – and ultimately our overall health – include the following:

Climbing the Mountain,[30] by lay apostle "Anne" and Bill Quinn, offers nine   concepts to growing spiritually to holiness. They are:

Love of neighbor

Love of God

Discouragement (dealing with)

Service to others

Joy in service

Love of Jesus

Love of the Divine Will

Unity with Jesus

Faith

"Anne" states *that Jesus told her "...each soul on earth has a path that has been traced out for him. His culture, his parents, and his placement in time, all of these things have been designed by Me. There are no separations in heaven so cultures and religions blend freely."* This does not mean there won't be crosses to bear in life on earth. *"Holiness is a process, and suffering is part of that process. It is all about service to heaven, in suffering, or in an absence of suffering,"* Jesus confirmed to "Anne."

Today, man is self-centered. Rather than thinking about service to heaven and people on earth, many are using their knowledge, gifts and talents for their own advancement. This is not how God intended us to live, according to "Anne" and Bill Quinn.

Pope John Paul II wrote many books. One of my favorites for spiritual development is In My Own Words.[31] Following are a few concepts and quotes from his book.

Materialistic concerns and one-sided values are never sufficient to fill the heart and mind of a human person. A life reduced to the sole dimension of possessions, of consumer goods, of temporal concerns will never let you discover and enjoy the fullness of your humanity. It is only in God –Jesus, God made man –that you will fully understand what you are. He will unveil to you the true greatness of yourselves.....

Prayer brings the saving power of Jesus Christ into the decisions and actions of everyday life. Be faithful to your daily prayers: they will keep your faith alive and vibrant. Prayer can truly change your life. For it turns your attention away from self and directs your mind and your heart toward the Lord. If we look only at ourselves, with our own limitations and sins, we quickly give way to sadness and discouragement. But if we keep our eyes fixed on the Lord, then our hearts are filled with hope, our minds are washed in the light of truth, and we come to know the fullness of the Gospel with all its promise and life….

People cannot live without love. They are called to love God and their neighbor… Hope comes from God, from our belief in God. People of hope are those who believe God created them for a purpose, and that he will provide for their needs. Inner peace comes from knowing that one is loved by God, and from the desire to respond to his love….

Much is to be envied of those who can give their lives for something greater than themselves in loving service to others….

We must not be afraid of the future. We must not be afraid of man. It is no accident that we are here. Each and every human person has been created in the 'image and likeness' of the One who is the origin of all that is. We have within us the capacities for wisdom and virtue….

You must put aside any fear in order to take Christ to the world in whatever you do—in marriage, as single people in the world, as students, as workers, as professional people. Christ wants to go to many places in the world, and to enter many hearts through you….

So, too, are we called to 'visit' the needs of the poor, the hungry, the homeless, those who are alone or ill.

The Pope wrote many other books that give additional perspectives on spirituality. <u>Crossing the Threshold of Hope</u>[32] is a great, international best seller, expressing his personal beliefs. He speaks with passion about ...*the existence of God, about the dignity of man, pain, suffering, evil, eternal life and the meaning of salvation, about hope, the relationship of Christianity to other faiths, and that of Catholicism to other branches of the Christian faith. His bottom line message is Be not afraid!*

Another bestseller is Tony Dungy's book, <u>Quiet Strength.</u>[33] Dungy is the former coach of the Indianapolis Colts. While in Indianapolis he won many division titles. In his book, he shares his tragedy of losing his eighteen- year-old son, and how he leaned on his faith. In his son's eulogy, he said, *God said in all things give praise to God.* (Philippians 4:6) He said that this is very hard to do during this type of tragedy. He said, however that he tries everyday to live his faith and teach others about integrity and character by his example. He said, ...*my journey is my faith, and there is life outside of football.* He claims he rests on the knowledge that *God knows what is best for those who love and serve the Lord.* (Romans 8:28) Dungy is an example of how responses to life and its challenges ultimately stem from faith, values and beliefs, and overwhelmingly affect our health.

In his book, <u>Freedom of Simplicity,</u>[34] author Richard J. Foster discusses how to live in simplicity by being disciplined. In his second book on spirituality, <u>Celebration of Discipline,</u>[35] he shares how to achieve that discipline. He addresses

Those are just a few of the spiritual resources available to aid in achieving the third Circle of Health, *"spirit is the life."*[1] as Edgar Cayce describes. In summary, look at beliefs and values as a way to grow deeper in spirituality, and to complete your Circle of Health.

The complete Circle of Health represents the physical, mental and spiritual aspects of our health, and is preventive in nature. Sometimes, despite all our best efforts to eat proper foods in the right combinations, to be aware of and practice the mind-body connection, and to be spiritually connected, we can't avoid illness. If that happens, the next section will assist us in our health care choices. There are many options available to us besides traditional medicines that include surgery, medication and radiation. Many complementary and natural health options remain to be explored.

PART FOUR

NATURAL HEALTH

This chapter will present multiple, alternative health care options that are available to us in addition to traditional medicine. As a Registered Nurse, I believe in integrating both areas of our health care system. As discussed in previous chapters, choices of foods, activity, lifestyle, and how we think all affect the outcomes in our Circle of Health. This quick reference guide summarizes a few of the many books available to us.

CHAPTER IX

Natural Health Care Options

Alternative Medicine, a Definitive Guide[25] by Deepak
Chopra, MD, is one of the best resources available for
explaining other therapies. Dr. Chopra's brief review of a
few of these therapies follows below:

1. Acupuncture *"...is based on the belief that health is
determined by a balanced flow of qi (or chi), the vital life energy
present in all living organisms."* Acupuncture theory professes
that *"...qi circulates in the body along 12 major energy pathways
called meridians, each linked to a specific internal organs and
organ systems....There are over 1,000 acupoints within the
meridian system that can be stimulated to enhance the flow of
qi. When special needles are inserted in to these acupoints just
under the skin, they help correct and rebalance the flow of energy,
and consequently relieve pain and restore health,"* Dr. Chopra
contends. *Acupuncture can also increase immune response
by balancing the flow of vital life energy throughout the body.
Chopra also believes that a wide variety of disease conditions can
be treated with acupuncture, from the common cold and flu, to
addiction and chronic fatigue syndrome, and is also effective as an
adjunct treatment for AIDS and some mental disorders.*

In Dr. Chopra's book, he discusses *auriculotherapy, or ear acupuncture. This therapy is based on the fact that certain points on the outer ear form a reflex system that can affect other areas when the points are properly stimulated. Paul Nogier, MD, found 30 basic auricular points used to treat pain, dyslexia, and other functional imbalances,* according to Chopra.

2. Applied kinesiology *incorporates the principles of a variety of holistic therapies, including chiropractic and osteopathic medicine, and acupuncture, "…and involves manual manipulation of the spine, extremities, and cranial bones as the structural basis of its procedures. An applied kinesiologist studies the activity of muscle and the relationship of muscle strength to health."* Applied kinesiology applies a simple strength resistance test on a specific muscle that is related to the organ or part of the body that is being tested. *"Because of the close clinical relationship between specific muscle dysfunction and related organ or gland dysfunction,"* Chopra asserts, *"applied kinesiology can be used to identify and treat a wide variety of health problems, whether the problem originates in a muscle, gland or organ."*

Chopra further says, *"The goals of applied kinesiology are to:*

Determine patient health status and correlate findings with standard diagnostic procedures, restore postural balances, correct gait impairment, improve range of motion, restore normal nerve function, achieve normal endocrine, immune, digestive and other internal organ functions, and intervene early in degenerative processes to prevent or delay pathological conditions."

According to Dr. Chopra, *"Applied kinesiology procedures are not intended as a single method of diagnosis. They should enhance standard diagnosis, and not replace it."*

3. Aromatherapy/Essential Oils *"is a unique branch of herbal medicine that utilizes the medicinal properties found in essential oils of various plants,"* according to Deepak Chopra, MD[25] *"...Aromatherapy uses essential oils to affect the body in several ways. The benefits of these oils can be obtained through inhalation, external application, or orally by ingestion,"* Chopra adds.

"The chemical makeup of essential oils gives them a host of desirable pharmacological properties, ranging from antibacterial, antiviral, and antispasmodic, to uses as diuretics (promoting production and excretion of urine), vasodilators (widening of blood vessels), and vasoconstrictors (narrowing blood vessels)," says Kurt Schnaubelt, PhD[25] *Essential oils also act on adrenal glands, ovaries, and the thyroid, and can energize or pacify, detoxify, and facilitate the digestive process,"* Schnaubelt continues. *"Essential oils, unlike pharmaceutical drugs, are in a complete and balanced form that our bodies are designed to absorb and use beneficially,"* states aromatherapist, Anne Vermilye, M.S., C.C.H.T., C.M.T.[25]

"Pure essential oils are expensive. It takes 1,000 pounds of plant to produce one pound of essence. This process involves manpower to cultivate and harvest the plant...," Schnaubelt says.[25]

It is expensive, but one or two drops go a long way. It's best to get it from a supplier. If not, the effectiveness of lower grade oils, or oils that are diluted, drastically diminishes over time due to a loss of the essential properties, Schnaubelt concludes.[25]

Following are some widely used essential oils that are used therapeutically, according to Dr. Schnaubelt and Anne Vermilye.[25]

Eucalyptus *is an antiviral and expectorant agents used as a diffuser, or topically as a chest rub for rheumatism, muscular pains or neuralgia.*

Everlast *is used by skin care professionals in dilutions of 2% or lower for tissue regenerating qualities on scars. Applied topically, it is a powerful anti-inflammatory agent and can prevent hemorrhaging and swelling after a sports injury or bruising.*

Geranium *is fragrant oil with antifungal and antiviral properties. It is gentle on the skin and provides the body with many fragrances of oil composition. (It has many applications including the treatment of endometriosis and menopausal problems, diabetes, throat diseases, blood disorders, acts as a sedative, etc.)[38]*

German Chamomile *is effective when used in the bath or in a massage oil blend. It can reduce a fever as it rids the body of bacteria.*

Ginger, *when used internally, relieves diarrhea, gas, and other digestive discomforts. A ginger/cardamom stomach pack applied externally soothes abdominal pain and tension.*

Lavender *is the classic oil for aromatherapy and has the broadest of benefits. It can be used undiluted on burns, scaldings, small injuries, skin ulcers, eczema, and insect bites.* (It has also been known to keep bed bugs away. Lavender's high ester content emits a calming and almost sedative-like quality. It has been used for mood and antidepressant properties.)[38]

Mandarin *has a calming property and universally pleasing fragrance, and is a top choice for releasing anxiety. It is typically dispersed in a room diffuser.*

Neroli *can be mixed with any carrier oil and a perfume or spray. It will ease anxiety and tension and menopausal upsets.*

Naiouli *calms respiratory allergies and is a vitalizing and balancing agent for overactive, oily skin. It helps with hemorrhoids (in the non-acute stage), and is also effective on bacterial and fungal infections.*

Palmarosa *has a pleasant fragrance and is an excellent antiseptic/ antiviral and has uses in skin care and in the treatment of herpes.*

Peppermint *is used to relieve nausea and travel sickness by placing a drop on the tongue. It is effective for irritable bowel syndrome. In France small doses of peppermint oil (50mg) are given three times a day as a liver stimulant during convalescence.* (It helps with joint pain, rheumatism, migraines, fatigue, toothaches, flu, and varicose veins, and, according to Valerie Worwood, it also keeps mice and fleas away.)[38]

Ravensara aromatica *is used as an inhalation remedy for bronchitis and respiratory infections. If applied topically, it can be used to treat shingles and other sores.*

Roman Chamomile *is recommended to calm an upset mind or body. A drop rubbed on the solar plexus can bring rapid relief of mental or physical stress. It may help with liver engorgement.* (It helps with insomnia. Beware of chamomile Maroc. It is not a true chamomile and cannot be used as such, according to Worwood. *"In general, Chamomile has antibacterial and anti-inflammatory properties and is used for burns, skin problems, asthma, hay fever, diarrhea, sprains, fever, strains and depressive states,"* she adds.)[38]

Rosemary has a variety of chemical oil compositions. The softest and most expensive type is **rosemary verbenon** used for skin care. It improves cell regeneration.[24] This is especially helpful on sore joints and muscles. It is a good physical and mental stimulant, as well as a good antiseptic. *"It can be used to treat muscle sprains, arthritis, rheumatism, depression, fatigue, memory loss, migraines, headaches, coughs, flu and diabetes,"* according to Worwood.[38]

Spikenard... *is often used at the core of aromatherapy blends that are aimed toward benefiting the psyche.*

Tea Tree *is a nonirritating antiseptic, and has antibacterial, antiviral and antifungal properties. Applied topically, it is useful in healing pustule-filled wounds or acne, and for treating many types of mild or chronic infections that occur in the mouth and genital area. (Worwood also claims that it can be used for athlete's foot, acne, ringworm, and toothaches.)*[38]

Thyme *is a powerful broad-spectrum antibiotic oil used to treat urinary infections and to eliminate parasites and Candida. It is best used internally, but is not recommended for daily use. (According to Worwood, thyme can also be used as a room diffuser in flu season, and it works wonders. It assists in eliminating toxins from the body, and helps with whooping cough, rheumatism,* *fatigue, and acne. It also discourages parasites and insects from invading your home.)[38]*

Essential oils can be combined for even better results. Eucalyptus radiata, ravensara aromatica, and niaouli on the skin after a shower help the body's resistance to sickness during the cold and flu seasons, according to Schnaubelt. Anise seed oil mixed with a spoon of honey, or by itself, relieves gastrointestinal cramping. Tarragon stimulates digestion and calms a nervous digestive tract. Energy can be enhanced with black spruce and peppermint oils, and is an effective stimulant that works by strengthening the adrenal cortex.[25]

<u>The Complete Book of Essential Oils and Aromatherapy</u> by Valerie Worwood[38] *recommends a basic kit of essential oils such as lavender, tea tree, peppermint, chamomile, eucalyptus, geranium, rosemary, thyme, lemon, and clove.*

We have already discussed all of those essential oils except for lemon and clove.

According to Dr. Worwood:[38]

*"**Lemon** has a tonic action on the lymphatic system and a stimulating action on the digestive system. It helps to maintain slimness, disperse cellulite, and keep wrinkles at bay."*

*"**Clove** is an antibacterial, antiseptic, and analgesic, and is good for the prevention of disease and infection. Toothaches, nausea, and digestive and muscular disorders respond quickly and positively with clove. Do not use undiluted on the skin. It has also been used to aid those with asthma and sinusitis, and as a sedative".*

I personally recommend Teu Fu oil for opening sinuses and the respiratory tract by breathing a drop from the cupped palms of your hands, inhaling through your nostrils, and exhaling slowly through your mouth.

4. **Biofeedback Training** *"is a method of learning how to consciously regulate bodily functions that are normally unconscious (such as breathing, heart rate, and blood pressure) in order to improve overall health. It refers to any process that measures and reports back information immediately about the biological system of the person being monitored,"* according to Patricia Norris, PhD in Chopra's book.[25] That information can then be used to influence body functions.

"Neurotherapy, also known as neurofeedback or brain-wave therapy, is a sophisticated form of biofeedback used to normalize and optimize brain-wave patterns (beta, alpha, theta, delta). This is accomplished through the use of a computerized system connected to electroencephalograph (EEG) sensors applied to the scalp...," continues Norris.[25] The computer rapidly analyzes the EEG readings. The brain is then encouraged to recognize normal healthy brain waves. *"Once the brain learns how to change its habitual wave patterns into those that are more appropriate for overall psychophysiological functioning,"* says Norris, *"the change tends to be permanent and often continues to improve even after treatment ends."*[25] This type of biofeedback has been helpful with *"stress and stress related disorders, including insomnia, TMJ syndrome, migraines, asthma, hypertension, gastrointestinal disorders and muscular dysfunction,"* Norris concludes.[25]

5. Body Work *"refers to a wide range of therapies such as massage, deep tissue manipulation, movement awareness, and bioenergetic therapies.... The benefits... include pain reduction, relief of musculoskeletal tension, improved blood and lymphatic circulation, and promoting deep relaxation."* [25]

According to Gertrude Beard, RN, R.P.T.,[25] *... the research studies on therapeutic effects of massage indicate that massage:*

Has a sedative effect upon the nervous system, and promotes voluntary muscle relaxation

Is effective in promoting recovery from fatigue produced by excessive exercise

Can help break up scar tissue and lessen fibrosis and adhesions, which develop from injury and immobilization

Can relieve certain types of pain

Provides effective treatment of chronic inflammatory conditions by increasing lymphatic circulation

Helps reduce swelling from fractures

Affects circulation through the capillaries, veins, and arteries, and increases blood flow through the muscle

Can loosen mucous and promote drainage of fluids from the lungs by using percussive and vibratory techniques

Can increase peristaltic action (muscular contractions) in the intestines to promote fecal elimination

According to Dr. Chopra,[25] *"Reflexology states that there are reflex areas in the hands and feet that correspond to every part of the body, including organs, and glands, and that these parts can be affected by stimulating the appropriate reflex areas. Reflexology is used to relieve stress and tension, stimulate deep relaxation, improve the blood supply, and promote the unblocking of nerve impulses to normalize and balance the entire body."*[25]

6. Cell Therapy, broadly speaking, *"...includes the use of human blood transfusions and bone marrow transplants as well as injections of cellular materials... to stimulate healing and treat a variety of degenerative diseases, such as arthritis, Parkinson's disease, atherosclerosis and cancer.*[25]

7. Chelation Therapy, as defined by Deepak Chopra, MD,[25] *"... is used to rid the body of unnecessary and toxic metals... and to improve circulation, helping reverse the process of atherosclerosis (hardening of the arteries). The reversal, when it occurs, is accomplished in part through the removal of the calcium content of plaque from the artery walls through the injection of chelating agents... can potentially help reverse atherosclerosis and prevents heart attacks and strokes... may be used as an alternative to bypass surgery remarkably increases energy.... It's performed on an outpatient basis, is painless, and takes approximately 3/1/2 hours. (For optimal results... doctors recommend an angioplasty) ... appears to provide a strong anti-aging effect, and takes 20-30 treatments at an average rate of 1-3 times per week."*

8. Chiropractic *"...focuses on the relationship between the structure of the spine and the function coordinated by the nervous system, and how this relationship affects the preservation and* *restoration of health."[25] It is safe and surgery- and drug-free. Millions of people have reported relief from back pain, asthma, headaches, hearing problems, and a long list of other illnesses. The goal of chiropractic medicine is to correct vertebral subluxations, and to allow the body to repair and to restore itself the way it was designed to do.*

9. Craniosacral Therapy *"manipulates the bones of the skull and the base of the spine and tailbone in order to treat a range of conditions, from headaches and ear infections to stroke, spinal cord injury, and cerebral palsy.... The craniosacral system has rhythmic motion... and the therapist monitors the wavelike motion to determine any restriction or dysfunction in the craniosacral system.... There are three major approaches to craniosacral therapy: sutural, meningeal and reflex."* [25]

10. Detoxification Therapy *"helps to rid the body of chemicals and pollutants and can facilitate a return to health.... As a result of the industrial revolution and the post- World War II petrochemical revolution, toxins have accumulated in the human system faster they can be eliminated. People now carry within their bodies a modern-day cocktail derived from industrial chemicals, pesticides, food additives, heavy metals (like lead), and anesthetics, plus the residues of pharmaceuticals, legal drugs (alcohol, tobacco, caffeine), and illegal drugs (heroin, cocaine, marijuana)."* [25] There are many forms of detoxification discussed in Dr. Chopra's book. One of the milder detoxifications is Tiao He Cleanse from Nature's Sunshine. The usual detox period is 15 days, but that can be extended to 30 days, and won't affect a person's daily routine.

11. *Energy Medicine* describes "...*both healing bioenergetic therapies and diagnostic screening devices used to measure the electromagnetic frequencies emitted by the body in order to detect imbalances that may be causing present illness or contributing to future disease.... Its premise is that both physical matter, including the human body, and the psychological processes (thoughts, feelings, attitudes) are expressions of energy.*"[25]

12. *Environmental Medicine* "*explores the role of dietary and environmental allergens in health and illness. Factors such as dust, molds, chemicals and certain foods may cause allergic reactions that can dramatically influence diseases ranging from asthma and hay fever to headaches and depression.*[25]

13. *Enzyme Therapy* uses "*... plant and pancreatic enzymes... in complementary ways to improve digestion and absorption of essential nutrients.... Enzymes are substances that make life possible,*" stated Edward Howell, MD "*No mineral, vitamin, or hormone can do any work without enzymes. They are the mutual workers that build the body from proteins, carbohydrates, and fats. The body may have the raw building materials, but without the workers, it cannot begin.*" [25]

14. *Flower Essences* "*directly address a person's emotional state to help facilitate both psychological and physiological well-being,* said Dr. Edward Bach.[25] "*By balancing negative feelings and stress, flower essences can remove emotional barriers to health and recovery. Behind all disease lies our fears, our anxieties, our greed, our likes and dislikes...True healing involves treating the very base of the cause of the suffering.*" This mind- body medicine *using flower essence "...allows people to be happy,"* Dr. Bach concludes.[25]

15. Guided Imagery uses *"...the power of the mind to evoke a positive physical response, reduce stress, slow heart rate, stimulate the immune system, and reduce pain."*[25] *"If you are a worrier,"* says Dr. Martin L. Rossman,[25] *"and especially if you ever worry yourself sick, you may be an especially good candidate for learning how to positively affect your health with guided imagery...."*[25]

16. Herbal Medicine, *"also known as botanical medicine or phytotherapy... has been used in all cultures throughout history... Approximately 25 % of all prescription drugs are derived from trees, shrubs, herbs... or plant extracts...,"* according to Dr. Chopra.[25]

"Modern medicine has veered away from use of pure herbs in its treatment of health disorders"... partly due to economics, says Dr. Chopra.[25] *"Herbs by their very nature cannot be patented....Drug companies cannot hold the exclusive right to sell a particular herb, and they are not motivated to invest in testing or promoting herbs,"* confirmed Dr. Chopra.[25] *The collection and preparation of herbal medicines cannot be as easily controlled as the manufacture of synthetic drugs, making profits less dependable. In addition, many of these medicinal plants grow only in the Amazonian rain forest or other politically and economically unstable places, which also affects the supply of the herb ... The scope of herbal medicine ranges from mild-acting plant medicines, such as chamomile and peppermint, to very potent ones such as foxglove from which the drug digoxin is derived.... There are an estimated 250,000 to 500,000 plants on the earth today, but*

only 5,000 have been extensively studied for their medicinal applications."[25]

"The word 'herb' in herbal medicine refers to a plant or plant part that is used to make medicine, spices, or aromatic oils for soaps and fragrances. An herb can be a leaf, flower, stem, seeds, root, fruit, bark, or any other plant part used for its medicinal, food flavoring, or fragrant property."[25]

Dr. Chopra[25] continues to describe the action of herbs as follows:

Adaptogenic …increases resistance and resilience to stress…

Alternative…gradually restores proper functioning of the body, increases health and vitality…

Anthelmintic…destroys or expels intestinal worms…

Anti- inflammatory…soothes or reduces inflammation in tissue…

Antimicrobial…helps the body destroy or resist pathogens…

Antispasmodic…eases cramps in various types of muscles…

Astringent…binds action on mucous membranes, skin, and other tissues… creates a barrier against infections, aids in healing wounds and burns…

Bitter…triggers the sensory response on the central nervous system with a variety of responses such as increased appetite and the flow of digestive juices, etc., and aids in liver detoxification…

Carminative…stimulates the digestive system to work properly through plants that are rich in aromatic oils…

Demulcent...soothes and protects inflamed tissues through herbs rich in mucilage, helps prevent diarrhea and reduces muscle spasms in the bowels...

Diuretic...increases the production and elimination of urine and waste...

Emmenagogue...stimulates menstrual flow...

Expectorant...stimulates mucous removal from the lungs...

Hepatic... tones and strengthens the liver, sometimes increases bile flow, facilitates digestion and removes toxins...

Hypotensive...lowers abnormal blood pressure...

Laxative...promotes bowel movements...

Nervine...helps the nervous system...

Stimulating...invigorates the physiological and metabolic activities of the body...

Tonic...nurtures and energizes, sometimes used as a preventative measure, frequently used in Chinese medicine...

Common herbs that possess some of the above traits are:[25]

Aloe Vera *for healing wounds and burns*

Bilberry *for circulatory and night vision improvements*

Cayenne Pepper *is a systemic stimulant, increases blood flow, and strengthens heartbeat and metabolic rates*

Chamomile used as an anti-inflammatory in gastrointestinal disorders, and assists in digestion - especially as an after-dinner drink

Chasteberry for hormonal imbalances in women

Devil's Claw for arthritic conditions that affect arms and legs and lower back pain, and stimulates appetite

Echinacea for wound healing, common cold, Multiple Sclerosis, respiratory and urinary tract disorders

Eleuthero for resisting and enduring stress, chronic gastritis, diabetes, hardening of the arteries, and the cell-attacking nature of cancer- fighting drugs

Ephedra for asthma and certain allergy medicines, has bronchodilator properties

Feverfew for menstrual difficulties, lowers fevers, and rheumatoid arthritis properties (antirheumatic properties)

Garlic for antibiotic, antifungal, and antiviral activities, clears congested lungs, helps prevent certain cancers, is a preventive measure for colds and flu, for intestinal worms, certain ulcers, gout, rheumatism

Ginger for improving digestion, nausea and motion sickness

Ginkgo Biloba for cerebral dysfunction, short term memory loss, dizziness, tinnitus, hearing loss due to circulation, and for heart and eye disorders, early stages of Alzheimer's-type dementia

Ginseng for coping with stress, has antioxidant, liver-protecting *and hypoglycemic effects, lowers blood cholesterol, and stimulates immune system, and aids in normalizing blood levels in Type II diabetes*

Goldenseal *for colds and upper respiratory infections, and digestive problems such as ulcers and colitis*

Hawthorn *for congestive heart failure, the cardiovascular system, hypotensive activities (lowering blood pressure), and as a sedative*

Hops *as a sleep aid - no dependence or withdrawal problems*

Horse Chestnut *for chronic venous insufficiency, lower leg swelling, nighttime leg cramps*

Kava- Kava *for anxiety - do not take if liver problems or jaundice occur, and for four weeks maximum*

Licorice *for peptic ulcers, gastritis, colic, bronchial problems, chronic hepatitis and cirrhosis, may produce sodium retention, not for those who are pregnant, hypertensive or have kidney disease*

Milk Thistle *for protection and prevention of many liver disorders – a liver tonic that shortens the course of liver hepatitis*

Nettle *for rheumatism, arthritis, hay fever, eczema, prostate and urinary tract problems, and as a safe diuretic*

Passion Flower *used as mild sedative for hypotensive properties and antispasmodic effects when combined with Hawthorn for digestive spasms from gastritis and colitis*

Peppermint *for digestive and bowel disorders, muscle and nerve pain and upper respiratory*

Pygeum *an anti-inflammatory reducing urinary symptoms related to benign prostatic hyperplasia (BPH)*

St. John's Wort *an anti- inflammatory, wound healing, mild sedative and pain reducing properties, for menopausal changes triggering irritability and anxiety, for mild depression - must be approved by physician if taking other medications*

Saw Palmento *for benign prostate hyperplasia (BPH)*

Senna *for stool softening with no adverse effects, does not cause dependence or alter electrolyte imbalance, should not be taken if pregnant or lactating*

Valerian *for nervousness that affects falling asleep, no major adverse reactions like other barbiturates*

Witch Hazel *for bleeding, easing of pain and swelling of hemorrhoids, swelling and varicose veins.* Go to www. edenfoods.com[6] for more information.

There are additional herbs recommended for household use as well.

- C herb for snake bites and bee stings

- Comfrey for respiratory congestion

- Capsicum for internal bleeding, especially at the onset of a stroke or heart attack

Bach Flower for emotional health based on the outcome of a designated assessment tool. For example, calming essence cream has five Bach flowers and a soothing effect on

emotions, muscle pain, sores, etc. Go to www.floweressence.
com[39] for more information.

Glyconutrients to be taken for as many months as the
number of years the problem has existed. See www.
mymannapages.com/susanhallnd.[13]

Blue Algae (Spirilina), and **Green Algae** have been known
to be used to boost immune systems <u>after</u> chemotherapy.
Vitamin C by mouth or through infusions and CoQ10
have also been known to boost immune system following
chemotherapy. (For more information, see <u>Killing Cancer</u>
<u>Without Killing Yourself</u> by Dr. Allen Chips) [40]

Teasel for nervous system problems and Multiple Sclerosis

NOTE: For ordering special herbs, see resource section in
back of book.

*17. **Homeopathy** " is a low cost, nontoxic system of medicine
used by hundreds of millions of people worldwide," asserts Dr.
Chopra.[25] "It is particularly effective in treating chronic illnesses
that fail to respond to conventional treatment and is also a superb
method of self-care for minor conditions such as the common cold
and flu…. The World Health Organization has cited homeopathy
as one of the systems of traditional medicine that should be
integrated world wide with conventional medicine in order to
provide adequate global care in the 21st century…."*

Homeopathy has three basic principles:[25]

*Like cures like (Law of Similars) - In large doses the same
substance produces the symptoms of an illness, but cures it in
minute doses (chicken pox, flu vaccine, measles, etc.).*

*The more a remedy is diluted, the greater its potency. (Some
experts also include titrated.)*

*An illness is specific to the individual. The physical, mental and
emotional symptoms are "profiled" to determine the best remedy or
combination of remedies based on personal symptoms.*

18. Hypnotherapy is another integrative option, according
to Dr. Chopra.[25] *"Hypnotherapy is used to manage numerous
medical and psychological problems. Hypnotic techniques can
help a person stop smoking, overcome alcohol and substance abuse,
and reduce overeating. Hypnotherapy is also effective for stress,
sleep disorders, and mental health problems such as anxiety, fear,
phobias and depression...The power of suggestion has played a
major role in healing in many cultures...."*

A misconception is that you may go into hypnosis
unwillingly. But, *"There can be no hypnosis unless the client is
willing to participate in the process. The client enters hypnosis in
a natural way, of his or her own accord, simply by following the
suggestions from the hypnotherapist."*[25]

The following hypnotherapy testimonial is relayed by Allen
Chips, D.C.H., PhD, [40] about one of his private practice
clients. *A young woman, who had been in a car accident, could
not be relieved of pain after years of constant traditional medical
interventions. As a last resort, she went to Dr. Chips, and was
hypnotized and taken back to the day of the accident. Her mind*

had told her body that her legs were chopped off in the car wreck. During the hypnotic state, an unusual healing occurred. When she woke up, she felt that something was different, and her pain was gone. X-rays showed that her legs were correctly aligned. The young woman said that when she went to the hypnotherapist, she recognized her legs as healed. The mother of this young lady is now a certified hypnotherapist, and has been asked to assist hospital patients. This is just one example of integrative medicine at its best, according to Dr. Chips.

19. Light Therapy *– "Light and color ... are sources of healing.... Results indicate that full- spectrum, ultraviolet, colored, and laser light can have therapeutic value for a range of conditions from chronic pain and depression, to immune disorders and cancer.... Melatonin, the chief hormone of the pineal gland, is produced only during darkness (its production is actually inhibited by light). Melatonin has sedative qualities and helps reduce anxiety, panic disorders and migraines, as well as inducing sleep. It has also been thought to be a primary regulator of the immune system.... There is mounting evidence that different colors of light have different effects on the body.... When light rays strike the retina of the eye, they are converted into nerve current, sometimes termed photocurrent.... Many people have a decreased level of photocurrent transmission...This condition – photocurrent deficit – can cause diminished brain function and can lead to numerous symptoms:*

Learning disability

Poor concentration and memory

Mental fogginess

Poor physical coordination and performance

Sleeping problems

Lack of self esteem

Mood swings

Seasonal affective disorder (SAD) or depression

Fear and anxiety

Hyperactivity

Fatigue

Headaches

Light sensitivity

Poor peripheral vision and night blindness[25]

20. Magnetic Field Therapy *"... can be used in both diagnosing and assisting in treatment of physical and emotional disorders. This process has been recognized to relieve symptoms and may, in some cases, retard the cycle of new disease. Magnets and electromagnetic therapy devices are now being used to eliminate pain, facilitate the healing of broken bones, and counter the effects of stress."*[25]

21. Naturopathic Medicine *"treats disease by utilizing the body's inherent ability to heal. Naturopathic physicians aid the healing process by incorporating a variety of options based* *on the patient's individualized needs. Diet, lifestyle, work and personal history are all considered when determining a treatment regimen.*"[25]

In Naturopathic Medicine, there are six time-tested principles:

"The healing power of nature ...."

"Treat the cause rather than the effect...."

"First, do no harm...."

"Treat the whole person..."

"The physician is a teacher ...who educates, empowers, and motivates patients to assume more personal responsibility for their own health...."

"Prevention is the best cure."

22. Neural Therapy *"...uses injections of anesthetics to remove short circuits in the body's electrical network. This process frees up the flow of energy and normalizes cellular function, making neural therapy an effective treatment for a variety of disease conditions, especially chronic pain...."*

"Conditions that normally respond to neural therapy include:

Allergies and asthma

Arthritis

Back pain and whiplash

Bladder dysfunction

Chronic pain

Colitis and ulcers

Depression

Dizziness

Ear problems

Emphysema

Headaches and migraines

Heart disease and circulatory disorders

Hemorrhoids

Hormonal imbalance

Glaucoma and inflammatory eye disease

Kidney and gall bladder disease

Liver disease

Menstrual cramps

Muscle and sports injuries

Post-operative recovery

Prostate disorders

Sinusitis

Skin disease

Thyroid dysfunction"[25]

23. Osteopathic Medicine *"…is a form of physical medicine that helps restore the structural balance of the musculoskeletal system. Combining joint manipulation, physical therapy, and postural reeducation, it is effective in treating spinal and joint difficulties, arteries, digestive disorders, menstrual problems, and chronic pain."*

24. Oxygen Therapy *"…alters the body's chemistry to help overcome disease, promote repair, and improve overall function. These therapies are effective for a wide variety of conditions, including infections (viral, fungal, parasitic, bacterial), circulatory problems, chronic fatigue syndrome, arthritis, allergies, cancer, and multiple sclerosis."*

25. Prolotherapy *"…rejuvenates the body by injection of natural substances to stimulate the growth of collagen to strengthen weak or damaged joints, tendons, ligaments, or muscles. It's cost-effective as an alternative to drugs and surgery for degenerative arthritis, low back pain, neck pain, joint pain, carpal tunnel syndrome, migraine headaches, and torn ligaments and cartilages."*

26. Qigong and Tai Chi *"…combine movement, meditation, and breath regulation to enhance the flow of vital energy in the body, improve circulation, and enhance immune function."*

27. Sound Therapy – *"Sound and music can have a very powerful effect on one's health. Sound therapy is used in hospitals, schools, corporate offices and psychological treatment programs as an effective treatment to reduce stress, lower blood pressure, alleviate pain, overcome learning disabilities, improve movement and balance, and promote endurance and strength."*

28. Yoga *"…is among the oldest known health practices in the* *world, and research into yoga has a strong impact on the fields of stress reduction, mind/body medicine, and energy medicine. The physical postures, breathing exercises, and meditation practices of yoga have proven to reduce stress, lower blood pressure, regulate heart rate, and even retard the aging process."*

More natural health care options exist such as Chinese medicine, orthomolecular medicine, NAET, natural hormone replacement therapy, longevity medicine, hyperthermia, hydrotherapy, guided imagery, etc. Explore all options to see what completes your Circle of Health. Remember, it took a lifetime for your body to evolve to its present condition. It takes at least 6-12 months to begin to see results from natural health approaches. Natural remedies sometimes take longer than synthetic products and traditional medicine, however, natural remedies may have fewer side effects on your overall health.

In addition to all those different therapies, a hair analysis should be done by your ND or MD to evaluate your body's responses to your environment and nutritional intake. This is a valuable tool for structuring your health care and, ultimately, in making the right choices for your body.

The next chapter discusses one of my patient's responses to food selections and combinations along with herbal supplements.

CHAPTER X

One Man's Journey

One of my clients shared his experience on his journey to a healthier lifestyle and, ultimately, to better overall health.

As a young person, Bill was very involved in athletics, participating in track, basketball, and football. When playing football in high school and college, he suffered many ankle and knee injuries.

In his late 20s, he tried running to stay healthy but ankle injuries interfered. In his 30s, he was active with his childrens' sports and coached their teams. His main exercise was walking at least three times a week. By the time he was 40, he was diagnosed with gout, and placed on medication. He also took medication to control chronic joint pain. In his late 40s, he was diagnosed with rheumatoid arthritis and placed on many medications to see what would work to control the pain.

Treatment to control rheumatoid arthritis included an injection that cost $1400 a month. Since his insurance did not cover this cost, he received assistance from the pharmaceutical company distributing this medication.

He is now in his mid-50s, and just recovered from prostate cancer after receiving radiation treatment and losing about 30 pounds. He remains about 20 pounds overweight, has high blood pressure, and reports great frustration at feeling sick, tired, and full of medications.

When he contracted the flu about one year ago, he stopped the injections for his rheumatoid arthritis. His doctor told him the shots compromise the immune system, exacerbating the flu's effects.

My client contacted me and I placed him on the following program, right after his 55th birthday:

Detoxification of his body – he chose a "Dieter's Cleanse" from Nature's Sunshine

No dairy products

No alcohol

No wheat, barley, amaranth, grains, or gluten products

No nightshade vegetables: tomatoes, green peppers, potatoes, mushrooms, eggplants

Add plant enzymes – he chose PDA from Nature's Sunshine

Add alfalfa – four capsules three times a day

Add una gato or cat's claw

Take two triple relief capsules three times a day from Nature's Sunshine

Take a multi vitamin or Trio vitamin from Nature's Sunshine

Add probiotics 11, taking four capsules for three days. Then chew two tablets of L. Reuteri for the next three days. Next, take four capsules of bifidophilus for the next three days. Repeat this routine over the next three months.

Take feverfew – two capsules three times a day

In addition, I gave him a chart of foods to eat for his "O" blood type.

After 30 days, he began to feel better. He had not received his injections for five weeks, surprising his rheumatologist. His doctor expressed concern about Bill's choice to curtail his injections, and ordered blood work. He told my client that eating right does not work for all rheumatoid arthritis clients. After completing a thorough assessment on my client, the doctor did not find any rheumatoid nodules. He did notice one bad ankle spot on my client and stated it was from uric acid. My client and his physician were pleasantly surprised when they received the lab report – the best results since Bill had become their patient.

When my client shared the results with me, I also ordered a hair analysis to confirm the results and to see if there were any other deficiencies. Tests showed that my client's zinc was low, so he added it to his daily supplements routine. He also added one extra vitamin C and D to boost his immune system.

He is now trying to take walks at least two to three times a week. He has eliminated the acute joint pain he experienced in the past when exercising. In 2008, when he had knee surgery for a torn meniscus, he asked me if there was anything else to alleviate that condition. I recommended Everflex, Super GLA, (Nature's Sunshine), Ole11, (Pure Herbs), and Glyconutrients, (Mannatech) which he decided to take. He also used essential oils, Theraroma Rheumatoid Rescue, and Theraroma Nerve-Ana extra strength. For his knee discomfort he used Joint Helper Natural Herbal roll on extra strength from Pure Herbs LTD. His goal is to put off knee surgery. Bill has now found that using the Reliv nutrional supplement products especially Arthoaffect that he has positive results in walking and his knee does not bother him as much in walking and in doing other activities.

My client stated that with those changes he could get up in the morning without joint pains and he could button a shirt. He felt that his quality of life had improved dramatically. He continues to make lifestyle adjustments and is committed to the diet since it has made a significant difference in his life. It has enabled him to remain essentially pain-free. It has been found that most rheumatoid arthritis patients suffer from food allergies. He does eat organic tomatoes occasionally with extra plant enzymes 22 and 27 from Nutritional Resources. He also plants a garden to provide home-grown foods.

He is still working with me, trying natural products for his blood pressure, and regularly consults with his doctor on his medications and health. He also stated that he has more energy and that he does not require naps as he had to have in the past. He is now looking forward to each day.

For more information on nutritional supplements refer to additional resources Reliv.com.

CHAPTER XI

Assessment Tools

Several assessment tools are used by naturopathic doctors. Three types addressed in this section are: iridology, muscle testing and hair analysis.

What is iridology? According to Peter Jackson-Main in his book, Practical Iridology,[41] it *"...is the examination and analysis of the colored portion of the eye, iris, in order to determine factors that may be important in the prevention and treatment of disease, as well as in the attainment of optimum health. One of the advantages of iridology is that it can reveal many aspects of an individual's health. An iris picture may suggest that where there is a problem, more than one organ may be involved, or that some emotional or mental element exists."* He continues by stating, *"Iridology affirms the uniqueness of each individual, and the power of the individual to manage his or her own health."* Remember, no two eyes are alike. This assessment assists in revealing what is right with you, and it can also show health issues that have occurred in the past. Iridology can guide you to a healthy lifestyle and help prevent diseases.

Peter Jackson-Main[41] further discusses constitution and

disposition of the eye. He states, *"Constitution is defined as the sum of your inherited and acquired characteristics..."* He adds, *"The three basic constitutional iris types consist of the two "pure" colors, blue (lymphatic) and brown (hematogenic), and the mixed iris."*

According to Jackson – Main,[41] the following are tendencies for each iris type:

Blue Iris:

Naturally adapted to a cooler climate

Prone to disturbances of the lymphatic system, the body's drainage network

Irritability of the mucous membranes, especially the upper respiratory tract, but also the gastrointestinal and urinary tracts and the skin

Raised acid levels, disturbances of kidney function

Rheumatic and allergic reactions

Easy onset of fever

Brown Iris:

Naturally adapted to a warm or hot climate

Disturbances of blood: thick blood, high blood fats, blood sugar abnormalities, mineral deficiencies

Disturbances of hormone activity (hormones are transported by the blood)

Tendency to excess (e.g. menstrual periods and crystalline deposits) and formation of stones and other accumulations

Hidden or "sub-acute" disease processes

Low reactivity, greater seriousness when fever does occur

Mixed Iris:

A blend of two distinct genetic sources

Tendency to disorders of the digestive system

Deficiency of digestive secretions from the liver, gallbladder, and pancreas

Can display characteristics of either lymphatic or hematogenic people, depending on the degree of pigmentation

There are many resources on iridology that discuss how to view and interpret the eye. (Refer to the eye chart in the appendix.) Peter Jackson –Main[41] also offers the following tips about reading eye charts. He states, *"When looking at the charts, remember it is as if you are looking at an individual, so the left eye will be to your right eye. The convention is to use positions of the clock to locate the organs, rather than degrees: top dead center of the iris is 12 o'clock or 0 minutes, opposite is 6 o'clock or 30 minutes."*

The next type of assessment tool is hair mineral analysis. This can be done by different laboratories. I utilize Trace Minerals Labs (TEI) in Texas. They have produced a booklet explaining the process called, *"Commonly Asked Questions about Hair Mineral Analysis"*.[42] The booklet says, *"...Your hair contains all the minerals present in your body, including nutritional minerals as well as toxic heavy metals. Hair mineral analysis is a laboratory test that measures this mineral content in the hair. It is very reliable and has a thousand references in peer-reviewed journals over the last 20 years.... There are 125 articles per week and over 6500 articles per year, not including the latest books and internet medical searches. The difference with blood and urine analysis is that these show what your levels are at the time of the test. Hair analysis measures storage levels over a period of time."*

In his book, <u>Trace Elements and Other Essential Nutrients</u>,[43] Dr. David Watts states, *"A hair sample, when properly obtained, analyzed, and interpreted, can provide information about one's metabolic and nutritional status. This includes the effect of diet, nutritional supplementation, stress, toxic metal exposure, and even inherited mineral patterns."* (Refer to the hair analysis sample in the index.)

The last assessment tool is referred to as kinesiology muscle testing. Barry LaPlante, LMBT, has held various workshops on this topic. He states in his article, "Your Body Doesn't Lie,"[44] that *"...your body is constantly receiving, processing, and responding to information from its internal and external environment. Developed forty years ago by Doctor Goodheart, applied kinesiology/muscle testing has become an invaluable clinical tool to help people regain their optimal health. Through extensive research, Dr. Goodheart found muscles actually weaken when introduced to different stress (food allergy, emotional stress, poor posture, trauma or injury.) During muscle testing certain points of your body are touched to assess your autonomic nervous system communication. This landmark discovery has spawned branches of kinesiology and research in this new and ever growing science around the globe,"* according to LaPlante .[44]

There are at least 45 applied kinesiology muscle testing points on our human body.   Dr. Patsy Reynolds, ND,[2] defines some of these points as: *blood pressure, protein, stress, pineal gland, allergies, sodium, lymphatic, thymus, stomach acid, liver, acidophilus, colon, zinc, vitamins A, B, C, D, E, F, magnesium, vitamin D, thyroid, pancreas, spleen, heart, carbohydrate, potassium, bladder, kidney, yeast, parasites, iron, enzymes, manganese, and adrenals.*

Those assessment tools utilized by naturopathic doctors present a holistic insight to your circle of health.

CONCLUSION

Start where you are now, and begin to build a healthier you. Think about food choices. Begin to look at the types of foods eaten. Are they acid or more alkaline? Gear choices to slightly alkaline foods such as fresh fruits and vegetables. Learn to eat until satisfied, not full. It is like filling the car with gas – do not overfill the tank.

Begin exercising now. Walk more. Add 30 minutes a day, working up to one hour. Keep moving and exercising and a fit body will be the result!

Take care of your mind. Feed it with positive thoughts and attitudes. Practice my mom's (Jane Chips) philosophy, "It's not what life throws you, but how you handle it that counts." After that, the most important area to work on is your spirituality. Your beliefs are the foundation for your health, life, and journey on this earth.

Remember: "Spirit is the life, mind is the builder, and the physical is the result."[1]

--Edgar Cayce

BOOKS AND WEBSITES

First Circle of Health

1. *Mind is the Builder, Your Life is the Result: Powerful Concepts from the Edgar Cayce Philosophy,* by Dick Daily, 3rd edition, 2006, A.R.E. Press, Virginia Beach, VA, pg. 9, reading 4722-1

2. Patsy Reynolds ND. Manns Harbor, drpatsy@pinn.net

3. Nature's Sunshine Products, Warsaw, IN, Product Catalog A-Z, 2008, www.nsp.com, 1-800-223-8225

4. American Holistic University, PO Box 7220, Kill Devil Hills, NC, 27948, (800) 296-MIND, www.AHUonline.org, Admissions@holistictree.com

5. Pure Herbs Company, 33410 Sterling ponds Blvd. Sterling, MI 48312, www.pureherbs.com

6. Kukicha Twig tea - www. Edentea.com

7. *Eat Right For Your Type,* by Dr. Peter J D'Adamo with Catherine Whitney, 1996, 1st Edition, G.P. Putnam's Sons, NY, Published by the Penguin Group, pgs. 54- 76, 95-120, 149-168, 188-208

8. *The Acid-Alkaline Diet,* by Christopher Vasey, ND, 2nd

Edition, 2006, Healing Arts Press, Rochester, VT

9. pH Health Assessment pamphlet, by Christopher Vasey, ND, 2007, pH ion Nutrition, Scottsdale, AZ

10. *Sick and Tired*, by Dr Robert Young and Shelly Young, 2001, Woodland Publishing, Pleasant Grove, UT, pgs. 31-37, 47, 55,57,61,63, 64-75

11. Nutritional Resources, www.phasesoftware.com, (1-800-867-7353)

12. *Choose Life or Death*, by Carey A. Reams with Cliff Dudley, 8th Edition, 2002, Holistic Wholesalers, LLC, Spencer, TN, pgs. 5, 145

13. *Mannatech Product Guide*, March ed. 2008, Coppell, Texas, www.mymannapages.com/susanhallnd

14. Sugars That Heal, by Emil I. Mondoa, MD, and Mindy Kitei, 1st Edition, Random House Publishing, NY

15. *The pH Miracle for Weight Loss*, by Robert Young and Shelly Young, 2005, Warner Wellness, NY and Boston, pg. 191

16. *pH Buffer*, Melbourne, FL, www.vaxa.com, (1-813-870-2904)

17. *Running on Empty: The Untold Truths*, by Dr. Alex Duarte, Edition 2006, Wasatch Research Institute, www.naturestool.com

18. *The Encyclopedia of Natural Healing*, by Siegfried Gursche MH, and Zoltan Rona, MD, MSc, and the Alive Research

Group, Second Edition, September 2002, Alive Publishing Group, Burnaby, BC Canada, pgs. 158-165

19. *Proper Food Combining Works*, by Lee DuBelle, 7th Edition, 1993, Walsh & Associates, Tempe AZ, pg. 43

20. *The Food Combining Guide*, by Wayne Pickering

21. *10 Essentials of Highly Healthy People*, by Walt Larimore, MD, 2003, Zondervan, Grand Rapids, MI, pgs. 31, 94-109, 75, 161, 165, 177, 179

22. Center for Disease Control, CDC.gov

23. *Encyclopedia of Natural Medicine*, by Michael Murray, ND, and Joseph Pizzorno, ND, 2nd Edition, 2002, Three Rivers Press, pg. 161

24. Fitness *for Dummies*, by Suzanne Schlosberg and Liz Neporent, MA, 3rd Edition, 2005, Wiley Publishing, Hoboken, NJ

Second Circle of Health

25. *Alternative Medicine: The Definitive Guide*, by Deepak Chopra, MD, 2002, Celestial Arts, Berkeley, CA, pgs. 1-465

26. *Stories the Feet Can Tell Thru Reflexology: Stories the Feet Have Told Thru Reflexology*, by Eunice Ingham, 10th Edition, 2005, Ingham Publishing, Inc., St Petersburg, FL, pgs. 97-100 and 27-29

27. *The Power of Your Subconscious Mind*, by Dr. Joseph Murphy, ed 2001, Bantum Books, NY, pgs 26-27

Third Circle of Health

28. *Your Best Life Now*, audio book by Joel Osteen, 1st Edition, 2007, Simon & Schuster, NY

29. *Become a Better You*, audio book by Joel Osteen, 1st Edition, 2004, NY Warner

30. *Climbing The Mountain – Discovering Your Path to Holiness*, by Anne and Bill Quinn, 2005, Directions for Our Times, Justice, IL

31. *In My Own Words*, by Pope John Paul II, 1st Edition,1998, Liguori, MO

32. *Crossing the Threshold of Hope*, by Pope John Paul II, 1st Edition, 2003, Alfred A. Knopf, NY

33. *Quiet Strength*, by Tony Dungy, 1st Edition, 2007, Tyndale House Publishers

34. *Freedom of Simplicity*, by Robert Foster, 1973, Harper Collins San Francisco, CA

35. *Celebration of Discipline*, by Robert Foster, Revised Edition, 1988, Harper Collins San Francisco, CA

36. *Words to Love By*, by Mother Teresa, 8th Edition, 1989, Ave Maria Press, Notre Dame, IN

37. Audio books and CDs by Joice Meyer: "The Cure for Stress"; "The Cause and Cure for Worry"; " Overcoming fear with Faith"; "Why do I Feel the Way I do"; "Contentment and Satisfaction", "Change"; Mind, Mouth, Moods, & Attitudes"; "*Eat the Cookie Buy the Shoes*", and many more...
Joyce Meyer Ministries, www.joycemeyer.org

Natural Health Care Options

38. *The Complete Book of Essential Oils and Aromatherapy*, by Valerie Ann Worwood, 1991, New World Library, San Rafael, CA, pgs. 19-22

39. www. Floweressence.com

40. *Killing Your Cancer Without Killing Yourself: Using Natural Cures...*, by Allen S. Chip,s DCH, PhD, 1st Edition, 2006, Transpersonal Publishing, Kill Devil Hills, NC, pgs. 46, 164

Assessment tools

41. *Practical Iridology,* by Peter Jackson-Main, 1st Edition, 2004, reprinted 2006, Carroll & Brown Publishers Limited, Queen's Park, London

42. *Commonly Asked Questions About Hair Analysis,* pamphlet by Trace Elements, Inc., Addison, TX 75001

43. *Trace Elements and Other Essential Nutrients,* by Dr. David L. Watts, 5th writer's block, 2006, Library of Congress catalog card no. 99-75783

44. *Your Body Doesn't Lie,* article by Barry LaPlante, LMBT, 2008, North Beach Sun

Additional Resources

Clinical Hypnotherapy: A Transpersonal Approach, by Dr. Allen Chips, DCH, Transpersonal Publishing, NC

Encyclopedia of Nutritional Supplements, by Michael T Murray, ND, Three Rivers Publishing, NY 2001

Medicinal Teas, www.InPursuitoOfTea.com

Herbal Products; www.drphil@HISgoodherbs.com, (770-252-7827)

Politics in Healing: The Suppression and Manipulation of American Medicine, by Daniel Haley

Hoxsey Therapy: When Natural Cancer Cures Became Illegal, by Harry Hoxsey, Transpersonal Publishing, NC

Biomedicalcenter (BMC) the Hoxsey Clinic, Ph (01152664) 684-9011, www.Hoxsey.com

National Association of Transpersonal Hypnotherapists, Hypnotherapy Training and Practitioners, 242-480-0530 or 1-800-296-MIND, www.holistictree.com

Perfect Balance- A natural medicine supplier with orasal, an anticancer enzyme, www.theperfectbalance.com, www.Salicinium.com

Immuno Augmentative Therapy (IAT) Clinic, Alternative Cancer Therapy clinic located in the Bahamas, www.immunemedicine.com

The Natural Health Bible, by Steven Bratman, MD, and David Kroll, PhD

The Complete Book of Enzyme Therapy, by Dr. Anthony J. Cichoke

Relive International, (nutritional therapies), St. Louis, MO, www.Reliv.com

Juice Plus+ Products drsusan@juiceplus.com

For further information regarding natural health
or nutritional support products and services,
contact the author or her business manager:

Susan Hall, RN, ND, PhD-----susanhallnd@yahoo.com
William Hall, Business Manager

TISSUE MINERAL ANALYSIS

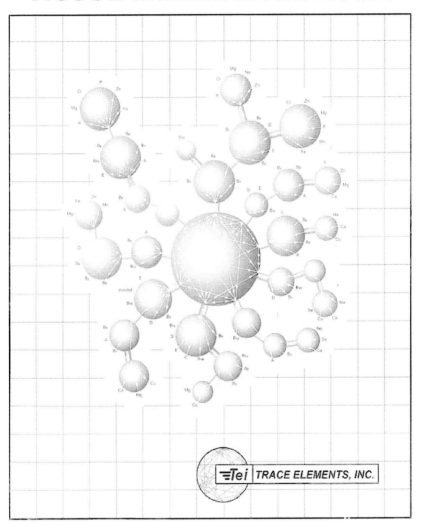

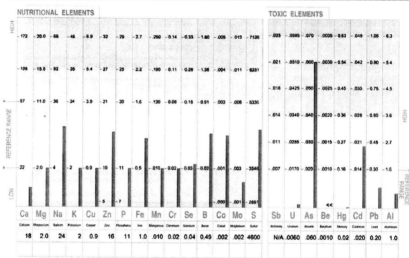

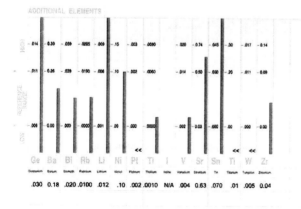

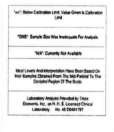

SIGNIFICANT RATIOS

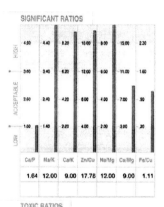

Ca/P	Na/K	Ca/K	Zn/Cu	Na/Mg	Ca/Mg	Fe/Cu
1.64	12.00	9.00	17.78	12.00	9.00	1.11

TOXIC RATIOS

Ca/Pb	Fe/Pb	Fe/Hg	Se/Hg	Zn/Cd	Zn/Hg	S/Hg	S/Cd	S/Pb
90.0	5.0	50.0	2.0	800.0	800.0	230000	230000	23000

ADDITIONAL RATIOS

	Current	Previous	
Ca/Sr	28.57		131/1
Cr/V	5.00		13/1
Cu/Mo	450.00		625/1
Fe/Co	500.00		440/1
K/Co	1000.00		2000/1
K/Li	166.67		2500/1
Mg/B	4.08		40/1
S/Cu	5111.11		1138/1
Se/Tl	40.00		37/1
Se/Sn	.57		0.67/1
Zn/Sn	228.57		167/1

LEVELS

All mineral levels are reported in milligrams percent (milligrams per one-hundred grams of hair). One milligram percent (mg%) is equal to ten parts per million (ppm).

NUTRITIONAL ELEMENTS

Extensively studied, the nutrient elements have been well defined and are considered essential for many biological functions in the human body. They play key roles in such metabolic processes as muscular activity, endocrine function, reproduction, skeletal integrity and overall development.

TOXIC ELEMENTS

The toxic elements or "heavy metals" are well-known for their interference upon normal biochemical function. They are commonly found in the environment and therefore are present to some degree, in all biological systems. However, these metals clearly pose a concern for toxicity when accumulation occurs to excess.

ADDITIONAL ELEMENTS

These elements are considered as possibly essential by the human body. Additional studies are being conducted to better define their requirements and amounts needed.

RATIOS

A calculated comparison of two elements to each other is called a ratio. To calculate a ratio value, the first mineral level is divided by the second mineral level.
EXAMPLE: A sodium (Na) test level of 24 mg% divided by a potassium (K) level of 10 mg% equals a Na/K ratio of 2.4 to 1.

SIGNIFICANT RATIOS

If the synergistic relationship (or ratio) between certain minerals in the body is disturbed, studies show that normal biological functions and metabolic activity can be adversely affected. Even at extremely low concentrations, the synergistic and/or antagonistic relationships between minerals still exist, which can indirectly affect metabolism.

TOXIC RATIOS

It is important to note that individuals with elevated toxic levels may not always exhibit clinical symptoms associated with those particular toxic minerals. However, research has shown that toxic minerals can also produce an antagonistic effect on various essential minerals eventually leading to disturbances in their metabolic utilization.

ADDITIONAL MINERALS

These ratios are being reported solely for the purpose of gathering research data. This information will then be used to help the attending health-care professional in evaluating their impact upon health.

REFERENCE RANGES

Generally, reference ranges should be considered as guidelines for comparison with the reported test values. These reference ranges have been statistically established from studying an international population of "healthy" individuals.
Important Note: The reference ranges should not be considered as absolute limits for determining deficiency, toxicity or acceptance.

INTRODUCTION TO HAIR TISSUE MINERAL ANALYSIS (HTMA)

Hair is used for mineral testing because of its very nature. Hair is formed from clusters of specialized cells that make up the hair follicle. During the growth phase the hair is exposed to the internal environment such as blood, lymph and extra-cellular fluids. As the hair continues to grow and reaches the surface of the skin its outer layers harden, locking in the metabolic products accumulated during the period of formation. This biological process provides a blueprint and lasting record of mineral status and nutritional metabolic activity that has occurred during this time.

The precise analytical method of determining the levels of minerals in the hair is a highly sophisticated technique; when performed to exacting standards and interpreted correctly, it may be used as a screening aid for determining mineral deficiencies, excesses, and/or imbalances. HTMA provides you and your healthcare professional with an economical and sensitive indicator of the long-term effects of diet, stress, toxic metal exposure and their effects on your mineral balance that is difficult to obtain through other clinical tests.

It is important for the attending healthcare professional to determine your mineral status as minerals are absolutely critical for life and abundant health. They are involved in and are necessary for cellular metabolism, structural support, nerve conduction, muscular activity, immune functions, anti-oxidant and endocrine activity, enzyme functions, water and acid/alkaline balance and even DNA function.

Many factors can affect mineral nutrition, such as: food preparation, dietary habits, genetic and metabolic disorders, disease, medications, stress, environmental factors, as well as exposure to heavy metals. Rarely does a single nutrient deficiency exist in a person today. Multiple nutritional imbalances however are quite common, contributing to an increased incidence of adverse health conditions. In fact, it is estimated that mild and sub-clinical nutritional imbalances are up to ten times more common than nutritional deficiency alone.

The laboratory test results and the comprehensive report that follows should not be construed as diagnostic. This analysis is provided only as an additional source of information to the attending doctor.

Test results were obtained by a licensed clinical laboratory adhering to analytical procedures that comply with governmental protocol and standards established by Trace Elements, Inc. U.S.A. The interpretive data based upon these results is defined by research conducted by David L. Watts, Ph.D.

UNDERSTANDING THE GRAPHICS

NUTRITIONAL ELEMENTS
This section of the cover page graphically displays the test results for each of the reported nutritional elements and how they compare to the established population reference range. Values that are above or below the reference range indicate a deviation from "normal". The more significant the deviation, the greater the possibility a deficiency or excess may be present.

TOXIC ELEMENTS
The toxic elements section displays the results for each of the reported toxic elements. It is preferable

that all levels be as low as possible and within the lower white section. Any test result that falls within the upper dark red areas should be considered as statistically significant, but not necessarily clinically significant. Further investigation may then be warranted to determine the possibility of actual clinical significance.

ADDITIONAL ELEMENTS

This section displays the results of additional elements for which there is limited documentation. These elements may be necessary for biochemical function and/or may adversely effect biochemical function. Further study will help to reveal their function, interrelationships and eventually their proper therapeutic application or treatment.

SIGNIFICANT RATIOS

The significant ratios section displays the important nutritional mineral relationships. This section consists of calculated values based on the respective elements. Mineral relationships (balance) is as important, if not more so, than the individual mineral levels. The ratios reflect the critical balance that must be constantly maintained between the minerals in the body.

TOXIC RATIOS

This section displays the relationships between the important nutritional elements and toxic metals. Each toxic metal ratio result should be in the white area of the graph, and the higher the better. Toxic ratios that fall within the darker red area may indicate an interference of that toxic metal upon the utilization of the nutritional element.

ADDITIONAL RATIOS

The additional ratios section provides calculated results on some additional mineral relationships. At this time, there is limited documentation regarding these ratios. For this reason, these ratios are only provided as an additional source of research information to the attending health-care professional.

METABOLIC TYPE

This section of the report will discuss the metabolic profile, which is based on research conducted by Dr. D. L. Watts. Each classification is established by evaluating the tissue mineral results and determining the degree to which the minerals may be associated with a stimulating and/or inhibiting effect upon the main "energy producing" endocrine glands. These glands regulate nutrient absorption, excretion, metabolic utilization, and incorporation into the tissues of the body: the skin, organs, bone, hair, and nails. How efficiently each nutrient is utilized depends largely upon proper functioning of the endocrine glands.

FAST METABOLISM (TYPE #2)

** Sympathetic Dominance
** Tendency Toward Decreased Thyroid Function (decreased secretion of hormones)
** Tendency Toward Increased Adrenal Activity (increased secretion of hormones)

The current mineral pattern is indicative of a fast metabolic rate (Fast Metabolism, Type #2). The glandular imbalance associated with Fast Metabolism (Type#2) is usually the result of an acute stress reaction or possible inflammatory condition. Type #2 Fast Metabolism is often associated with high energy. However, energy levels may fluctuate particularly when under stress. It should be noted that stress is a normal part of life and serves a useful purpose when it is controlled. However, chronic uncontrolled stress will eventually contribute to various vitamin and mineral imbalances, and the ability to maintain adequate energy levels and optimum health will decrease.

NUTRIENT MINERAL LEVELS

This section of the report may discuss those nutritional mineral levels that reveal moderate or significant deviations from normal. The light blue area's of each graph section represent the reference range for each element based upon statistical analysis of apparently healthy individuals. The following section, however, is based upon clinical data, therefore an element that is moderately outside the reference range may not be commented on unless determined to be clinically significant.

NOTE:
For those elements whose levels are within the normal range, it should be noted that nutritional status is also dependent upon their critical balance with other essential nutrients. If applicable, discussion regarding their involvement in metabolism may be found in the ratio section(s) of this report.

CALCIUM (Ca)
The tissue calcium level is below the normal level. This is not uncommon for this age and fast metabolism (Type #2). However, if this profile worsens or continues for an extended period of time, a tendency toward experiencing one or more of the following symptoms will increase:

Anxiety	Insomnia
Allergies	Dental Problems
Irritability	Muscle Cramps
Aggressiveness	Mood Swings

SOME FACTORS THAT MAY CONTRIBUTE TO A LOW TISSUE CALCIUM LEVEL
* Increased Adrenal Activity
* Hypoparathyroid Activity
* Excess Phosphorus Retention
* Toxic Metal Accumulation
* Inadequate Calcium Intake

MAGNESIUM AND PARATHYROID HORMONE
Magnesium, along with calcium regulates the synthesis and/or release of parathyroid hormone. Together, low tissue levels of magnesium and calcium may be indicative of decreased parathyroid activity, which can result in decreased calcium and magnesium absorption from the diet.

MANGANESE (Mn) AND BLOOD SUGAR REGULATION
The mineral manganese in combination with certain vitamins and minerals is essential for many biochemical reactions, including carbohydrate metabolism and energy production. Manganese deficiency is frequently related to such manifestations as, low blood sugar levels, ligamentous problems and reproductive dysfunction.

GERMANIUM (Ge)

Your germanium level of 0.03 mg% is above the established reference range for this element. Excessive intake of germanium has been reported to adversely affect kidney function and cause disturbance in skeletal muscle function. Long-term intake of germanium has been reported to cause:

Anemia	Weight Loss
Neuropathy	Myopathy
Autonomic Dysfunction	Nerve Palsies
Kidney Dysfunction	Vomiting

HERBAL SOURCES OF GERMANIUM

Some herbs naturally contain significant levels of germanium. At this time, the following herbs should be discontinued if presently being consumed.

Garlic	Aloe
Comfrey	Ginseng
Watercress	Chlorella
Reishi Mushrooms	Shiitake Mushrooms

LITHIUM (Li)

Although your lithium level is moderately elevated, it should not be considered as clinically significant at this time. However, if a disturbance between this element and another mineral exists, clinical significance may be noted in the appropriate ratio section of this report.

TIN (Sn)

Your tin level of 0.07 mg% is above the established reference range. It has been reported that an excessive level of tin can interfere with iron metabolism and will produce heme breakdown. Elevated tin also increases the excretion of selenium and zinc from the body.

SOME SOURCES OF TIN

Canned Foods	Dental Fillings
Herbs	PVC
Fungicides	
Dental Treatments	Stannous Fluoride
Toothpaste	Marine Paints
Cooking Utensils	Collapsible Metal Containers
Solders	Mining

NUTRIENT MINERAL RATIOS

This section of the report will discuss those nutritional mineral ratios that reveal moderate or significant deviations from normal.

Continuing research indicates that metabolic dysfunction occur not necessarily as a result of a deficiency or excess of a particular mineral level, but more frequently from an abnormal balance (ratio) between the minerals. Due to this complex interrelationship between the minerals, it is extremely important that imbalances be determined. Once these imbalances are identified, corrective therapy may then be used to help

NAME: SAMPLE, SUSIE

re-establish a more normal biochemical balance.

NOTE: The "Nutritional Graphic" developed by researchers at Trace Elements, and presented on the cover of this report shows the antagonistic relationships between the significant nutrients, including the elements (arrows indicate antagonistic effect upon absorption and retention).

HIGH SODIUM/POTASSIUM (Na/K) RATIO AND STRESS

Stress produces an indirect affect upon your body's mineral patterns. The body responds to stress by increasing and/or decreasing the release of certain hormones from the endocrine glands. The hormones in turn will influence the body's absorption, retention and excretion of nutrients, including the minerals. The early stage of stress is known as the alarm stage, and the hormones initiating an alarm reaction will produce an increase in sodium retention relative to potassium. Therefore, this pattern is indicative of the alarm stage of stress. This pattern may also be associated with an inflammatory reaction or increased histamine production.

HIGH ZINC/COPPER (Zn/Cu) RATIO

The zinc level is high relative to tissue copper status (see high Zn/Cu ratio). A low copper level in conjunction with a zinc-copper imbalance is a strong indicator of a decrease in the role of copper in many functions of metabolism. One of the basic functions of copper is its necessity in collagen synthesis. If this profile becomes both severe and chronic, a decrease in collagen synthesis can occur. This can then be a precurser to capillary fragility, bleeding gums, osteoporosis and premature greying of the hair.

HIGH SODIUM/MAGNESIUM (Na/Mg) RATIO

The sodium level is high relative to magnesium (see high Na/Mg ratio). These two minerals should be in balance (4.2/1), and when sodium is excessive relative to magnesium, there is frequently an increase in magnesium requirements.

MAGNESIUM AND ASTHMA

Low magnesium intake has been found in groups of people experiencing lung problems such as wheezing and asthma. Histamines can trigger lung problems and are also known to increase the requirement for magnesium.

TOXIC METAL LEVELS

Hair is used as one of the tissue's of choice by the Environmental Protection Agency in determining toxic metal exposure. A 1980 report from the E.P.A. stated that human hair can be effectively used for biological monitoring of the highest priority toxic metals. This report confirmed the findings of other studies which concluded that human hair may be a more appropriate tissue than blood or urine for studying community exposure to some trace metals.

A heavy metal may be elevated in this HTMA and yet no known environmental exposure can be ascertained at this time. This is not unusual, as exposure may have originated years earlier. Additionally, research has found that heavy metals can be inherited by the fetus during pregnancy. Heavy metals can be found in the body for years following the original exposure and will remain in body tissues until removal is initiated. For example, the half-life of cadmium in some tissues will range from ten to thirty years.

ARSENIC (As)

NAME: SAMPLE, SUSIE

Your arsenic level of 0.06 mg% is above the established reference range. Arsenic has been found high in some seafood obtained from coastal waters, particularly shrimp, oysters, and mussles. Other sources include arsenic rich soils, herbicides, arsenic containing insect sprays, burning of arsenate treated building materials in fireplaces, coal combustion, and smelters.

CADMIUM (Cd)

The cadmium level is within the cautionary range. The following are some fairly common sources of cadmium:

Tobacco	Zinc Smelters
Burning Plastics	Galvanized Water Pipes
Superphosphate Fertilizers	Auto Exhaust
Electronics Industry	

NOTE:

At this time, further confirmation of heavy metal toxicity using a blood test may or may not reveal an elevated level. This is due to the protective response of the body, in which following a toxic metal exposure, the element is sequestered from the blood and stored in various other tissues. Therefore, if the exposure is not ongoing or chronic, elevated levels in the blood may not be present. It is recommended that another analysis be performed in at least one year to monitor any changes in toxic metal accumulation.

TOXIC METAL RATIOS

ALL CURRENT TOXIC METAL RATIOS ARE WITHIN THE ACCEPTABLE RANGE

DIETARY SUGGESTIONS

The following dietary suggestions are defined by several factors: the individual's mineral levels, ratios and metabolic type, as well as the nutrient value of each food including protein, carbohydrate, fat, and vitamin and mineral content. Based upon these determinations, it may be suggested that foods be avoided or increased temporarily in the diet to aid in the improvement of your biochemistry.

GENERAL DIETARY GUIDELINES FOR THE FAST METABOLIZER

* INCREASE INTAKE OF HIGH PURINE PROTEIN FOODS...high purine protein sources include liver, kidney and heart. Other good sources include sardines, tuna, clams, crab, lobster and oysters. Unless notified otherwise, high purine and moderate purine protein intake should constitute approximately 33% of total daily caloric intake.

* INCREASE INTAKE OF MILK AND MILK PRODUCTS...such as cheese, yogurt, cream, butter (unsalted). Increase intake of nuts and seeds such as almonds, walnuts, peanuts, peanut butter and sunflower seeds. Foods high in fat unless notified otherwise should constitute approximately 33% of total daily caloric intake.

* REDUCE CARBOHYDRATE INTAKE...including unrefined carbohydrates. Sources such as cereals, whole

- 6 -

grains and whole grain products are contraindicated for frequent consumption until the next evaluation. Carbohydrate intake in the form of unrefined carbohydrates should be approximately 33% of total daily caloric intake.

* AVOID ALL SUGARS AND REFINED CARBOHYDRATES...this includes white and brown sugar, honey, candy, soda pop, cake, pastries, alcohol and white bread.

FOOD ALLERGIES

In some individuals, certain foods can produce a maladaptive or "allergic-like" reaction commonly called "food allergies". Consumption of foods that one is sensitive to can bring about reactions ranging from drowsiness to hyperactivity in children, itching and rashes, headaches, high-blood pressure and arthritic pain.

Sensitivity to foods can develop due to biochemical (nutritional) imbalances, and which stress, pollution, and medications can aggravate. Nutritional imbalance can further be contributed to by restricting food variety, such as eating only a small group of foods on a daily basis. Often a person will develop a craving for the food they are most sensitive to and may eat the same food or food group more than once a day.

The following section may contain foods that are recommended to avoid. These foods should be considered as potential "allergy foods", or as foods that may impede a rapid and effective reponse. Consumption of these foods should be avoided completely for four days. Afterwhich, they should not be eaten more frequently than once every three days during course of therapy.

FOODS THAT STIMULATE HISTAMINES

Consumption of the following foods can stimulate histamine release in certain metabolic types and may contribute to respiratory-type allergy reactions. These foods are to be avoided until the next evaluation or until notified otherwise by attending doctor.

Beet Greens	Rhubarb
Apples	Chocolate
Spinach	Black Tea
Eggplant	Strawberries
Sweet Potatoes	Peanuts
Blueberries	Green Beans
Pecans	Chard
Wheat Germ	Concord Grapes
Cocoa	Collards
Parsley	Blackberries
Beets	

FOODS HIGH IN MAGNESIUM

The following foods are high in magnesium content relative to calcium and sodium. These foods may be increased in the diet until the next evaluation.

Blackstrap Molasses	Corn
Prunes	Cashews
Avocados	Wild Rice
Bananas	Tofu
Bass (broil)	Garbanzo Beans
Figs (dried)	

THE FOLLOWING FOODS MAY BE INCREASED IN THE DIET UNTIL THE NEXT EVALUATION

Mozzarella Cheese	Turnip Greens
Milk	Mustard Greens

Kale	Yogurt
Monterey Cheese	Cream
Almonds	Buttermilk
Swiss Cheese	

HIGH COPPER FOODS TO INCREASE IN THE DIET

The following foods are good sources of dietary copper. If desired, these foods may be increased in the diet until the next evaluation.

Cod	Lobster
Brazil Nuts	Mushrooms
Pecans	Crab
Hazelnuts	Almonds
Pistachio Nuts	Sesame Seeds
Sunflower Seeds	Walnuts
Duck	Liver

AMINO ACIDS THAT IMPROVE CALCIUM ABSORPTION

Calcium absorption is greatly enhanced when the diet is high in the amino acids, lysine, arginine and histadine. These proteins also help to reduce acidity of the tissues. Both effects are favorable for the fast metabolizer, therefore addition of any of the following foods to the diet is recommended at this time:

Lima Beans	Soybeans
Garbanzo Beans	Sausage (lean)
Rumproast	Lamb
Skim Milk	Smelt
Beef Stew	Vegetable Stew
Cottage Cheese	Canadian bacon
Spare Ribs	Peanuts
Lentils	Bass
Flounder	Heart
Cod	Chuck Roast
Ham	Liverwurst
Salami	

SPECIAL NOTE

This report contains only a limited number of foods to avoid or to increase in the diet. FOR THOSE FOODS NOT SPECIFICALLY INCLUDED IN THIS SECTION, CONTINUED CONSUMPTION ON A MODERATE BASIS IS ACCEPTABLE UNLESS RECOMMENDED OTHERWISE BY YOUR DOCTOR. Under some circumstances, dietary recommendations may list the same food item in the "TO EAT" and the "TO AVOID" categories at the same time. In these rare cases, always follow the avoid recommendation.

CONCLUSION

This report can provide a unique insight into nutritional biochemistry. The recommendations contained within are specifically designed according to metabolic type, mineral status, age, and sex. Additional recommendations may be based upon other supporting clinical data as determined by the attending health-care professional.

OBJECTIVE OF THE PROGRAM:

The purpose of this program is to re-establish a normal balance of body chemistry through individually designed dietary and supplement suggestions. Properly followed, this may then enhance the ability of the body to more efficiently utilize the nutrients that are consumed, resulting in improved energy production and health.

REMOVAL OF HEAVY METALS:

Re-establishing a homeostatic balance or equilibrium of body chemistry will enhance the body's ability to remove heavy metals naturally. The elimination of a heavy metal involves an intricate process of attachment of the metal to proteins, removal from storage areas, and transport to the eliminative organs for excretion. Improvement in ones nutritional balance will improve the capability of the body to perform these tasks and eliminate toxins more easily.

However, the mobilization and elimination of metals may cause temporary discomfort. As an example, if an excess accumulation of iron or lead is contributing to arthritic symptoms, a temporary flare-up of the condition may occur from time to time. This discomfort can be expected until removal of the excess metal is complete.

Your Circle of Health

DIET SUMMARY PAGE

This page may be removed from the HTMA Report and used as a quick-reference dietary guide. As this is solely a summary page, please refer to the dietary portion of the report to obtain more detailed information on why a particular food item is listed in the "Foods To Avoid" or "Foods That May Be Increased" section. For those foods that are not specifically mentioned below, continued consumption on a moderate basis is acceptable unless recommended otherwise by the attending healthcare professional.

FOODS TO AVOID UNTIL THE NEXT EVALUATION

Alcohol	Apples	Beans - Green	Beet Greens
Beets	Blackberries	Blueberries	Bread - White
Cakes	Candy	Chard	Chocolate
Cocoa	Collards	Eggplant	Grapes - Concord
Honey	Parsley	Pecans	Peanuts
Rhubarb	Soda	Spinach	Strawberries
Sugar	Sweet Potatoes	Tea - Black	Wheat Germ

FOODS THAT MAY BE INCREASED IN THE DIET

Almonds	Avocados	Bacon - Canadian	Bananas
Bass	Bass - Broiled	Beans - Garbanzo	Beans - Lima
Beef - Stew	Brazil Nuts	Buttermilk	Cashews
Cheese - Cottage	Cheese - Monterey	Cheese - Mozzarella	Cheese - Swiss
Clams	Cod	Corn	Crab
Cream	Duck	Figs - Dried	Flounder - Baked
Ham	Hazelnuts	Kale	Lamb
Lentils	Liverwurst	Lobster	Milk - Skim
Milk - Whole	Molasses - Blackstrap	Mushrooms	Mustard Greens
Oysters	Peas	Pistachio Nuts	Prunes
Rice - Wild	Roast - Chuck	Roast - Rump	Salami
Sausage - Lean	Sesame Seeds	Smelt	Sunflower Seeds
Tofu	Tuna	Turnip Greens	Vegetable Stew
Walnuts	Yogurt		

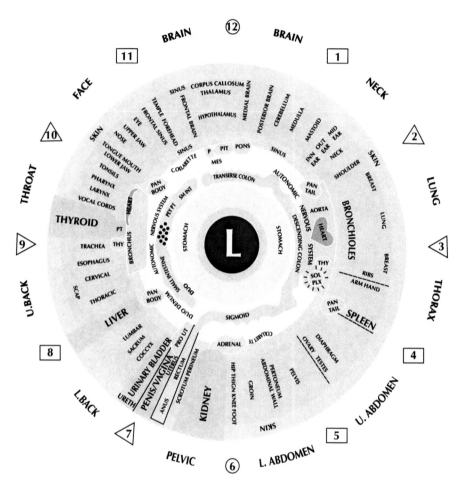

Abbreviations:
HF: Hepatic Flexure
PRO: Prostate,
PEY PT: Peyers Patches
P: Pineal
PT: Parathyroid

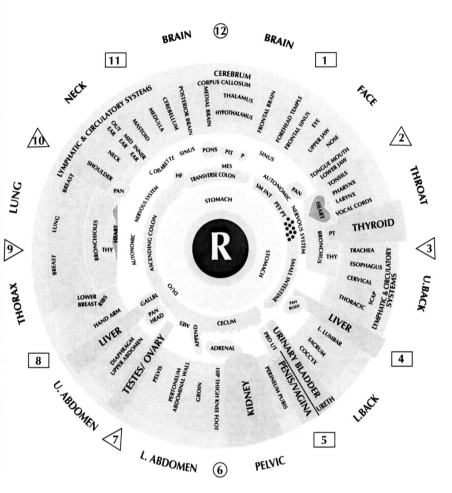

Abbreviations:
HF: Hepatic Flexure
PRO: Prostate,
PEY PT: Peyers Patches
P: Pineal
PT: Parathyroid

Other Books by
Transpersonal Publishing

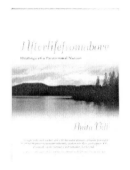

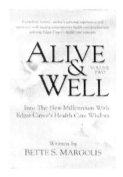

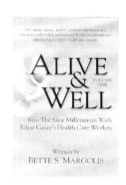

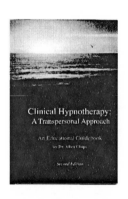

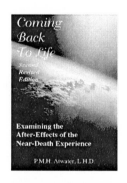

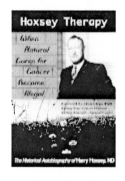

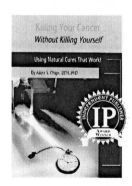

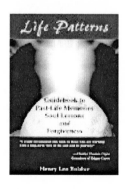

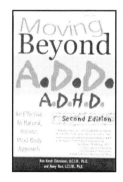

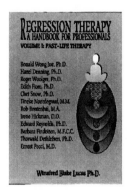

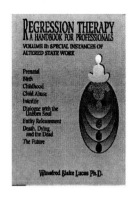

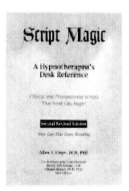

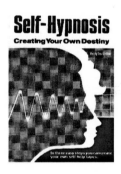

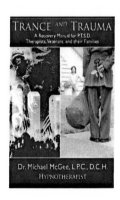

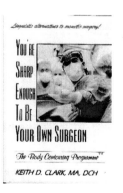

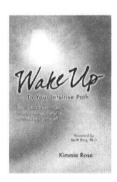

To see these and other books by the publisher, go to:
www.TranspersonalPublishing.com